Sports Injury Care

Thomas E. Abdenour, ATC
Athletic Trainer
Golden State Warriors

Alton L. Thygerson, Ed.D., EMT
Consultant, First Aid Institute
National Safety Council

JONES AND BARTLETT PUBLISHERS
BOSTON   LONDON

Editorial, Sales, and Customer Service Offices

Jones and Bartlett Publishers
One Exeter Plaza
Boston, MA 02116
617-859-3900
1-800-832-0034

Jones and Bartlett Publishers International
7 Melrose Terrace
London W6 7RL
England

Production Editor: Natasha Sabath
Editorial and Production Service: Publication Services, Inc.
Cover Design: Hannus Design Associates
Prepress, Printing and binding: Haddon Craftsmen

Library of Congress Cataloging-in-Publication Data

Sports injury care / Thomas E. Abdenour & Alton L. Thygerson
    p. cm.
Includes bibliographical references.
ISBN 0-86720-282-3
1. Sports—medicine and supplies.   2. Physical education and training—medical services.   I. Abdenour, Thomas E.   II. Title.
GV745.W35   1992
796'.028—dc20   92-13401
                                                                         CIP

Printed in the United States of America
97 96 95   10 9 8 7 6 5 4 3

CONTENTS

FOREWORD

As a head coach in the NBA since 1976, I have been repeatedly blessed with a front row seat for a run of sold-out performances starring the world's greatest athletes. In recent years our league has enjoyed a meteoric rise in both popularity and viability. Superstars like Julius Erving, Larry Bird, Magic Johnson, and Michael Jordan have led the way, with the enlightened support of commissioner David Stern, the NBA Board of Governors, and the NBA Players Association.

A great deal of credit should also go to the dedicated professionals who specialize in sports medicine. These are the people who keep our players healthy and able to perform at peak levels. This hard work continues to advance the quality of our games and interest in our sport to new heights.

I believe that Tom Abdenour, athletic trainer for the Golden State Warriors since 1987, is one of the best in his field. Whether you are an athlete, parent, coach, or trainer, I encourage you to use this carefully prepared book as a comprehensive guide to a better understanding of sports injuries.

In closing, please allow me to remind you that all the games we play, the important one being the game of life, are meant to be enjoyed. Don't be afraid to ask for the help of a doctor or a professional trainer when it's needed, because if you stubbornly insist on playing in pain, you are really playing in vain.

Wishing you good health and great fun!

Don Nelson
Head Coach and General Manager
Golden State Warriors

INTRODUCTION

Think back to when you have seen a sports injury. With the exception of college and professional teams, the coach is usually the first person to see and treat an injured athlete. Since there is usually no physician or other medically trained personnel around, the coach is responsible for giving immediate care. Later, the coach will have to decide whether the injured athlete can return to play or should receive medical care.

If the team or school has an athletic trainer or a physician, that expert's advice should be sought. But how many schools have these people at every game or practice? Moreover, how many nonschool teams have a trainer or a physician? Only if these teams have the son or daughter of a trainer or physician participating are they likely to have ready access to either.

Therefore, people expect coaches to have the answers. Fortunately, most sports injuries do not threaten life, nor are they severe. But there is always the possibility that a severe, life-threatening injury can occur at any level of athletic endeavor. Parents look to coaches for direction when their children are injured. It is not enough for a coach to simply say, "I don't know." A coach should either have the answer or know how to get the answer quickly. Legal expectations exist, too. A coach is responsible for caring for his or her athletes' injuries.

Often, care for a sports injury begins at home. The injured athlete may never have mentioned his or her injury to the coach, who could have done something about it if he or she had known. The athlete may not think the injury amounts to much or may keep quiet about it for fear of being benched. So it will be up to a parent to provide the care for the injury and to seek any needed medical attention.

Some athletes "go it alone," since injuries happen during participation in individual sports and activities at which no coach is present. Parental help may also be missing if the athlete is not living at home.

Sports injuries demand that someone make a decision about the proper care for the injured athlete. This book helps in such decision making with its decision-table (if . . ., then . . . table) format. Decision tables not only help identify what may be wrong (the "if" part of the decision table), but also help determine what to do about it (the "then" part of the table).

The following table shows estimates of the number of participants and injuries associated with various sports. Because this list is not complete and the number of participants varies greatly, no inference should be made concerning the relative hazard of these sports with respect to risk of injury. But the table points out that a lot of athletes get injured.

Sport	Participants	Injuries	Sport	Participants	Injuries
Archery	5,600,000	3,696	Ice hockey	1,500,000	31,342
Baseball	15,400,000	321,806	Ice skating	7,000,000	23,443
Basketball	26,200,000	486,920	Racquetball	8,200,000	13,795
Bicycle riding	56,900,000	514,738	Roller skating	21,500,000	74,994
Billiards	29,600,000	4,153	Skateboarding	7,500,000	65,819
Bowling	40,800,000	17,351	Snowmobiling	(*)	9,985
Boxing	(*)	4,546	Soccer	11,200,000	101,946
Fishing	46,500,000	65,677	Swimming	70,500,000	65,757
Football	14,700,000	319,157	Table tennis	13,700,000	1,732
Golf	23,200,000	24,224	Tennis	18,800,000	22,507
Gymnastics	(*)	34,383	Volleyball	25,100,000	92,961
Handball	(*)	3,942	Water skiing	10,800,000	21,499
Horseback riding	10,100,000	46,928	Wrestling	(*)	36,428

Source: Participants — National Sporting Goods Association (1989); figures include those who participate more than one time per year except for bicycle riding and swimming, which include only those who participate more than six times per year. Injuries — Consumer Product Safety Commission (1989); figures include only hospital emergency room treated injuries.   *Data not available.   Source: National Safety Council; *Accident Facts*, 1991.

A predictable risk of injury in sports exists. The older and bigger the athlete, the greater the risk for injury. After puberty, the chance for contact and collision increases, and the greater the severity of the injury.

Contact sports have higher injury rates than noncontact sports. Although boys are injured at twice the rate of girls, rates are similar if contact sports (in which boys participate more than girls) are eliminated.

Legal Concerns	Because physicians, athletic trainers, and emergency medical technicians are scarce at games and practices, the law requires a coach to provide first aid.

Paid employment as a coach requires the administration of first aid to an injured athlete. However, because of the relationship which exists between a coach and the injured athlete, even unpaid volunteers are required to render first aid. In other words, all coaches must give first aid to any injured athlete he or she is coaching.

Coaches have been sued. For example, in *Duda v. Gaines*, a coach was held negligent for not seeking immediate attention for a football player's dislocated shoulder. Rather than understanding the complications of such an injury, the coach reduced the shoulder, only to have it again dislocate, with further joint damage, three days later.

Emergency information cards should be maintained for all athletes. These information cards should include a consent-for-treatment form signed by parents. The cards should also contain the names of the athlete's physician and health insurance company. These cards should be kept available for use at all times in order to prevent medical treatment delays.

Whether you are a coach, parent, athletic trainer, or even an individual caring for yourself, this guide provides a quick, useful reference to turn to when the inevitable sports injury occurs.

1

Assessing the Injured Athlete and Checking for Shock

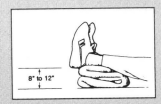

Assessment is the cornerstone of good injury care. The first goal in assessment is to determine all life-threatening conditions and, if needed, start resuscitation. Next, all conditions needing attention prior to moving the athlete must be addressed. Some conditions require calling the emergency medical services (EMS) system or, if thought safe, transporting the injured athlete without the use of an ambulance.

During the assessment, you should be careful not to move the athlete any more than necessary. Any unnecessary movement or rough handling should be avoided because it might aggravate undetected fractures or spinal injuries.

An assessment is divided into two parts:
- *Primary survey* for life-threatening conditions
- *Secondary survey* for nonemergency conditions.

Primary Survey

The *primary survey* tries to find and correct life-threatening conditions. Most of the time the primary survey will be completed quickly since most injured athletes you will see do not have life-threatening conditions.

If the primary survey uncovers any problems, such as an obstructed airway or massive bleeding, you must attend to them immediately before proceeding with the rest of the victim assessment.

The primary survey steps can be remembered by using the acronym **ABC$_2$DE:**

A—*Airway open?* If the athlete is talking or is conscious, the airway is open. For an unconscious athlete open the airway with the head-tilt/chin-lift method—unless a neck injury is suspected. See page 20 for more information.

B—*Breathing?* Conscious athletes are breathing. However, note any breathing difficulties or unusual breathing sounds. If the athlete is unconscious, keep the airway open and *look* for the chest to rise and fall, *listen* for breathing, and *feel* for air coming out of the athlete's nose and mouth. See page 21 for more information.

C$_2$—*Circulation?*
1. Check circulation by feeling for a pulse at the side of the neck (carotid artery). If a pulse is absent, cardiopulmonary resuscitation (CPR) is required. See page 24 for more information.
2. Check for severe bleeding by looking over the athlete's entire body for blood (blood-soaked clothing and/or blood pooling on the floor or ground). Bleeding requires the application of direct pressure (could use a pressure bandage). See pages 37–38 for more information.

D—*Disability?* Once the airway, breathing, and circulation have been assessed, you can determine the athlete's level of consciousness to see if there is any obvious central nervous system (CNS) damage. Whenever forceful trauma has happened, always suspect a spinal injury and stabilize until EMS personnel arrive. The athlete's level of consciousness or "mental status" can be quickly described by using one of the following classifications. It can be determined by following the simple acronym *AVPU,* which stands for:

   A—*Alert.* Eyes open and the athlete can answer questions in a clear manner. He or she knows their phone number, where they are, and their own name.

   V—*Verbal stimulus response.* Eyes do *not* open, and the athlete may not know his or her phone number. They may not know where they are, or their own name, but they do respond in some meaningful way when spoken to.

   P—*Painful stimulus response.* Eyes do *not* open and the athlete does *not* respond to verbal questions. Athlete responds to pinching of the skin.

   U—*Unresponsive.* The athlete does *not* respond to pinching of the skin.

E—*Expose and Examine.* Clothing may be hiding an injury or a severe bleeding site. How much clothing should be removed varies, depending on what conditions or injuries are found. The general rule is to remove as much clothing as necessary in order to determine the presence or absence of a condition or injury.

Secondary Survey	After completing the primary survey and attending to any life-threatening problems it uncovers, continue making an assessment called the *secondary survey*. This survey will discover injuries and/or conditions which do not pose an immediate threat to life, but which may do so if they remain undetected and uncorrected. Even minor injuries need treatment.

Rely on the acronym **CHECK** which stands for:

C—*Chief complaint and cause.* Athlete's answer when you ask "What's wrong?" or "Where do you hurt?" is called the chief complaint. Also find out what happened.

H—*History.* Attempt to find out what medical problems the athlete has that may be causing the athlete's condition and what information about these problems should be passed on to medical personnel. Ask about: (a) allergies, (b) medications, and (c) past health problems.

E—*Exact location.* Gently touch, feel, or probe the injury site for any obvious or unusual deformity.

C—*Compare.* If possible, compare the injured area with the same area on the opposite side of the body to determine anything unusual.

K—*Keep monitoring the athlete for change in his or her condition and keep a written record of what you find.* This will help a physician, should one be needed, with a later diagnosis.

Once the secondary survey is completed, you will know about the athlete's injury(ies) and/or condition. You can then systematically treat the injury(ies) and/or condition.

Checklist for Assessing the Injured Athlete	**Primary Survey: ABC$_2$DE**
	A—Airway open?
	B—Breathing?
	C$_2$—Circulation?
	1. Check circulation by feeling carotid (neck) pulse
	2. Check for severe bleeding

D—Disability?
   A—Alert
   V—Verbal stimulus response
   P—Painful stimulus response
   U—Unresponsive
E—Expose and examine

Secondary Survey: CHECK

C—Chief complaint and cause
H—History (preexisting medical problems)
E—Exact location
C—Compare
K—Keep monitoring and keep written record

Checking for Shock   The first hour after a serious injury is the most critical because of the danger of the athlete going into shock. The way you respond to an emergency situation could make the difference between life and death.

Shock occurs when the body cannot keep enough blood going to the vital organs, such as the brain, heart, and lungs. Every injury affects the circulatory system to some degree, and so first aid for shock should always be given—even before any signs of shock appear.

Many different types of shock exist; the type associated with trauma is known as hypovolemic shock.

Shock

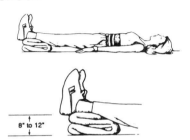

If injured athlete has . . .	THEN . . .
• become restless and nervous • a rapid pulse • cold and clammy skin • complained of thirst and is sweaty • a pale or blue face • rapid breathing • complained of nausea	1. Call the emergency medical services (EMS) system (usually 9-1-1). 2. If a spinal injury is suspected, do not move the athlete. 3. Check for and maintain a clear airway and breathing. 4. Control bleeding (usually direct pressure is sufficient). 5. Raise the legs 8 to 12 inches (keep legs straight). Do not raise legs if they may be fractured. 6. Splint broken bones. 7. Avoid rough handling of the athlete.

S
H
O
C
K

Shock (continued)

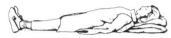

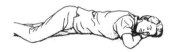

If injured athlete has . . .	THEN . . .
	8. Put blankets under and on top of the athlete.
	9. If possible, keep the athlete flat on his or her back. Exceptions are:
	—head injured (elevate head and shoulders)
	—stroke victim (elevate head and shoulders)
	—unconscious (keep on side)
	—vomiting (keep on left side)
	—breathing difficulties and/or chest injured (keep in semisitting position)
	—heart attack (keep in semisitting position).
	10. Do not give the athlete anything to eat or drink.

S
H
O
C
K

Emergency Medical Services (EMS) System

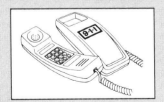

The emergency medical services (EMS) system consists of several components:
- first responders (law enforcement agency or fire service member or others designated in industry, government, and the private sector)
- EMS dispatcher located at the local emergency communications center
- emergency medical technicians with various levels of training working with well-equipped emergency vehicles
- hospital emergency department staff (e.g., physicians, nurses).

EMS Telephone Numbers

Activate the EMS system by using:
- 9-1-1 (covers the majority of people in the United States)
- seven-digit local number found on the inside front cover of the telephone directory
- 0 (zero or operator) as a last resort if unable to use the other numbers.

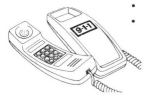

What Information to Give?	Give to the EMS dispatcher:

- **The athlete's location.** Give address, names of intersecting streets or roads and other landmarks if possible.
- **Your phone number.** This prevents false calls, and allows the center to call back for additional information if needed.
- **What happened.** Tell the nature of the emergency (e.g., heart attack, drowning, etc.).
- **Number of persons needing help and any special conditions. What is the athlete's condition** (e.g., conscious, breathing, etc.) **and what is being done for the athlete** (tell about CPR, rescue breathing).

Always hang up the phone last!

Basic Life Support*
(CPR and Choking Management)

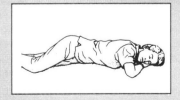

*Based on the 1992 American Heart Association guidelines for cardiopulmonary resuscitation and emergency cardiac care.

When to Start CPR?	You need to be able to:

When to Start CPR?

You need to be able to:
- recognize the signs of no breathing and no heartbeat
- provide first aid for breathlessness and pulselessness
- call for the emergency medical services (EMS).

Athletes who suffer a heart attack have a good chance of surviving if:
- CPR is started within the first 4 minutes of heart stoppage
- they receive advanced cardiac life support within the next 4 minutes.

Brain damage begins after 4–6 minutes and is certain after 10 minutes when no CPR is given.

Disease Precautions

Hepatitis B virus
- causes serious liver disease
- is very infectious.

AIDS:
- kills all HIV-infected victims
- presently has no cure.

Whenever possible, while giving CPR:

- cover open wounds with dressings or waterproof material (e.g., plastic wrap) to prevent contact with the blood
- use disposable latex gloves
- use a clear plastic face mask or shield with a one-way valve during rescue breathing.

The U.S. Centers for Disease Control report no evidence of transmission of either hepatitis B virus or AIDS during mouth-to-mouth resuscitation on CPR manikins or humans.

Signs of Successful CPR

Successful CPR refers to correct CPR performance, not survival of the athlete. Even with successful CPR, most stricken athletes will not survive unless they receive advanced cardiac life support (e.g., defibrillation, oxygen, and drug therapy). CPR serves as a holding action until such medical care can be provided. Early bystander CPR (started in less than 4 minutes after cardiac arrest) coupled with an EMS system with advanced cardiac life support capability (within 8 minutes) can increase the chances for survival to more than 40%.

Check CPR's effectiveness by:

- watching chest rise and fall with each rescue breath
- checking pulse after first minute of CPR and every few minutes afterward to determine if a pulse has returned
- having a second rescuer feel for carotid pulse while giving chest compressions. A pulse should be felt each time a compression is made. If alone, do not try to give compressions with one hand while checking for a pulse at the same time.

What about the Athlete's Clothing?

- Usually it's not necessary to remove or loosen athlete's clothing.
- Remove or loosen clothing if:
  —collar does not allow you to feel the carotid pulse
  —heavy clothing does not allow you to locate the notch at the tip of the sternum
  —you are unable to find correct hand position
  —your locale allows EMS personnel to remove all of an athlete's clothing, or any protective equipment that is in the way—by cutting, ripping, or pulling it up—in order to bare the chest. This includes either cutting a woman's bra or slipping it up to her neck.

Rescue Breathing and CPR

STEP	ACTION
1	**If you see a motionless athlete**
	Check responsiveness
	• If head or neck injury is suspected, move only if absolutely necessary.
	• Tap or gently shake athlete's shoulder.
	• Shout near athlete's ear, "Are you OK?"
2	**Activate EMS system.**

Rescue Breathing and CPR (continued)

STEP	ACTION
3	**Roll athlete onto back** Gently roll athlete's head, body, and legs over at the same time. Do this without further injuring the athlete.
4	**Open the athlete's airway** (use head-tilt/chin-lift method) • Place hand nearest athlete's head on athlete's forehead and apply backward pressure to tilt head back. • Place fingers of other hand under bony part of jaw near chin and lift. Avoid pressing on soft tissues under jaw. • Tilt head backward without closing athlete's mouth. • Do *not* use your thumb to lift the chin.

C
P
R

Rescue Breathing and CPR (continued)

STEP	ACTION
4 (continued)	**If you suspect a neck injury** Do *not* move athlete's head or neck. First try lifting chin without tilting head back. If breaths do not go in, slowly and gently bend the head back until breaths can go in.
5	**Check for breathing** (take 3–5 seconds) • Place your ear over athlete's mouth and nose while keeping airway open. • *Look* at athlete's chest to check for rise and fall; *listen* and *feel* for breathing.

Rescue Breathing and CPR (continued)

STEP	ACTION
6	**Give 2 full breaths** • Keep head tilted back with head-tilt/chin-lift to keep airway open. • Pinch nose shut. • Take a deep breath and seal your lips tightly around athlete's mouth. • Give 2 full breaths, each lasting 1½ to 2 seconds (you should take a breath after each breath is given to athlete). • Watch chest rise to see if your breaths go in. • Allow for chest deflation after each breath. **If neither of these 2 breaths went in** Retilt the head and try 2 more breaths. If still unsuccessful, suspect choking, also known as foreign body airway obstruction (see *Unconscious Adult Foreign Body Airway Obstruction* below).

C
P
R

STEP	ACTION
7	**Check for pulse** • Maintain head-tilt with hand nearest head on forehead. • Locate Adam's apple with 2 or 3 fingers of hand nearest athlete's feet. • Slide your fingers down into groove of neck on side closest to you (do not use your thumb because you may feel your own pulse). • Feel for carotid pulse (take 5–10 seconds). Carotid artery is used because it lies close to the heart and is accessible. **If there is a pulse** Give rescue breaths (mouth-to-mouth resuscitation) every 5 seconds. Every minute, stop and check the pulse for 5 to 10 seconds to make sure there is still a pulse.

C
P
R

Rescue Breathing and CPR (continued)

STEP	ACTION
7 (continued)	Continue until: • Athlete starts breathing on his or her own OR • Trained help, such as emergency medical technicians (EMTs), arrive and relieve you OR • You are completely exhausted. **If there is no pulse** If you are trained in CPR (cardiopulmonary resuscitation), you should stop every minute and check for a pulse for 5 to 10 seconds. Give CPR until: • Victim revives OR • Trained help, such as emergency medical technicians (EMTs), arrive and relieve you OR • You are completely exhausted.

C
P
R

Rescue Breathing and CPR (continued)

STEP	ACTION
7 (continued)	If you are not CPR trained, try to: 1. Get help from bystanders who might be trained. 2. Call the local emergency telephone number (usually 9-1-1). Often the dispatcher can give instructions about how to perform CPR.

Conscious Adult Foreign Body Airway Obstruction (Choking)

STEP	ACTION
1	**If athlete is conscious and cannot speak, breathe, or cough . . .** **Give up to 5 abdominal thrusts** (Heimlich maneuver) • Stand behind the athlete. • Wrap your arms around athlete's waist. • Make a fist with 1 hand and place the thumb side just above athlete's navel and well below the tip of the sternum. • Grasp fist with your other hand. • Press fist into athlete's abdomen with quick upward thrust. • Each thrust should be a separate and distinct effort to dislodge the object. After every 5 abdominal thrusts, check the victim and your techniques.

C
P
R

Conscious Adult Foreign Body Airway Obstruction (Choking) (continued)

STEP	ACTION
2	**Repeat cycles of up to 5 abdominal thrusts until:** • athlete coughs up object, or • athlete starts to breathe or cough forcefully, or • athlete becomes unconscious (use methods for an unconscious victim), or • you are relieved by EMS or other trained person.

Unconscious Adult Foreign Body Airway Obstruction (Choking)

STEP	ACTION
1	**If person is unconscious and breaths have <u>not</u> gone in . . .** **Give up to 5 abdominal thrusts** (Heimlich maneuver): • Straddle athlete's thighs. • Put heel of one hand against middle of athlete's abdomen slightly above navel and well below sternum's notch (fingers of hand should point toward athlete's head). • Put other hand directly on top of first hand. • Press inward and upward using both hands with up to 5 quick abdominal thrusts. • Each thrust should be distinct and a real attempt made to relieve the airway obstruction. Keep heel of hand in contact with abdomen between abdominal thrusts.

C
P
R

Unconscious Adult Foreign Body Airway Obstruction (Choking) (continued)

STEP	ACTION
2	**Perform finger sweep** • Use only on an unconscious athlete. In a conscious athlete, it may cause gagging or vomiting. • Use your thumb and fingers to grasp athlete's jaw and tongue and lift upward to pull tongue away from back of throat and away from foreign object. • If unable to open mouth to perform the tongue-jaw lift, use the crossed-finger method by crossing the index finger and thumb and pushing the teeth apart. • With index finger of your other hand, slide finger down along the inside of one cheek deeply into mouth and use a hooking action across to other cheek to remove foreign object.
	If the above steps are unsuccessful Cycle through the following steps in rapid sequence until the object is expelled or EMS arrives: • 2 rescue breaths, retilt head, 2 more breaths • up to 5 abdominal thrusts • finger sweep.

| How to Remember the Basic Life Support Steps | *Basic Life Support for an Adult Victim* |

R Responsive?

A Activate the EMS system (usually call 9-1-1).

P Position victim on back

A Airway open (use head-tilt/chin-lift or jaw thrust)

B Breathing check (look, listen, and feel for 3–5 seconds)
- If breathing and spinal injury not suspected, place in recovery position
- If not breathing, give 2 slow breaths; watch chest rise
  —If 2 breaths go in proceed to step C
  —If 2 breaths did not go in, retilt head and try 2 more breaths
  —If second 2 breaths did not go in, give 5 abdominal thrusts; perform tongue-jaw lift followed by a finger sweep; give 2 breaths, retilt head followed by 2 more breaths. Repeat thrusts, sweep, breaths sequence

C Circulation check (at carotid pulse for 5–10 seconds)
- If there is a pulse, but no breathing give rescue breathing (1 breath every 5–6 seconds)
- If there is no pulse, give CPR (cycles of 15 chest compressions followed by 2 breaths)

After 1 minute (4 cycles of CPR or 10–12 breaths of rescue breathing), check pulse.
- If no pulse, give CPR (15:2 cycles) starting with check compressions
- If there is a pulse but no breathing, give rescue breathing.

Basic Life Support for a Child or Infant Victim

E   Establish unresponsive

S   Send bystander, if available, to activate the EMS system (usually call 9-1-1).

P   Position victim on back

A   Airway open (use head-tilt/chin-lift or jaw thrust)

B   Breathing check (look, listen, and feel for 3–5 seconds)
- If breathing and spinal injury not suspected, place in recovery position
- If not breathing, give 2 slow breaths; watch chest rise
  - —If 2 breaths go in proceed to step **C**
  - —If 2 breaths did not go in, retilt head and try 2 more breaths
  - —If second 2 breaths did not go in, then . . .

  For a child: give 5 abdominal thrusts; perform tongue-jaw lift and if object is seen perform a finger sweep; give 2 breaths, retilt head followed by 2 more breaths. Repeat thrusts, mouth check, breaths sequence

  For an infant: give 5 back blows and 5 chest thrusts; perform tongue-jaw lift and if object is seen perform a finger sweep; give 2 breaths, retilt head followed by 2 more breaths. Repeat blows, thrusts, mouth check, breaths.

Basic Life Support for a Child or Infant Victim (continued)

C   Circulation check (for 5–10 seconds)
   • *For a child:* at carotid pulse   *For an infant:* at brachial pulse
   • If there is a pulse, but no breathing give rescue breathing (1 breath every 3 seconds)
   • If there is no pulse, give CPR (cycles of 5 chest compressions followed by 1 breath)

After 1 minute (10 cycles of CPR or 20 breaths of rescue breathing), check pulse.
   • If alone, activate the EMS system
   • If no pulse, give CPR (5:1 cycles) starting with check compressions
   • If there is a pulse but no breathing, give rescue breathing.

4

Open Wound Care

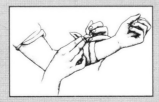

| **Open Wounds** | An open wound is a break in the skin. |

Types of open wounds:

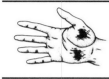

a. **Abrasion** (also known as floor or mat burn, artificial "rug" burn, skinned knee or elbow, strawberry, scrape)—scraping away of the first layer of skin; limited bleeding.

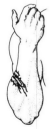

b. **Incision**—cut with smooth edges; bleeds freely.

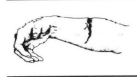 c. **Laceration**—cut with jagged edges; bleeds freely.

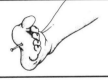 d. **Puncture**—pointed object penetrates skin and causes small hole.

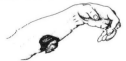 e. **Avulsion**—skin flap is torn loose or pulled off.

Open Wound Care

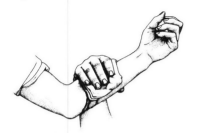

IF ..	THEN
open wound exists	Treat the open wound by: • controlling bleeding • preventing infection • stopping/reducing pain. To accomplish these goals: 1. Expose wound site. 2. Wash your hands in a vigorous scrubbing action with soap and water if available. If unavailable, use an alcohol wipe.

Open Wound Care (continued)

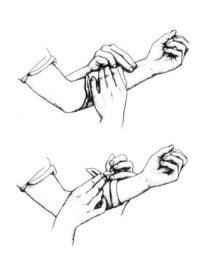

IF . . .	THEN . . .
open wound exists	3. Stop bleeding by: —applying direct pressure over wound using a sterile gauze. Protect yourself by using disposable latex gloves if contact may be made with athlete's blood or body fluids. **OR** —holding sterile gauze pad over wound with bandage applying the pressure (i.e., roller gauze). Do not remove a blood-soaked dressing since clots may be disrupted and bleeding may start again. Place new dressings on top of the blood-soaked ones.

W
O
U
N
D
S

Open Wound Care (continued)

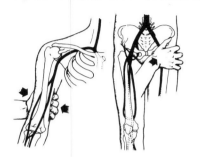

IF . . .	THEN . . .
open wound exists	**OR** —holding sterile gauze over wound and elevating the injured part at the same time. Do *not* elevate a broken extremity. **OR** —using pressure points while still applying direct pressure over wound. Using pressure points requires a skillful first aider. Unless exact location of the pulse point is known, the pressure point method is useless. Two locations on both sides of body may be used: (1) brachial point in the arm and (2) femoral point in the groin.

WOUNDS

Open Wound Care (continued)

IF . . .	THEN . . .
open wound exists	4. Clean wound with soap and water. Irrigate wound with ample water under pressure. —Wash the skin about 2 inches around the wound site to kill germs. —Do *not* wash deep or large wounds or those with bleeding that is difficult to control. Dress and bandage wound and have a physician cleanse wound. —Cuts deeper than $\frac{1}{8}$ inch or longer than $\frac{1}{2}$ inch, or those involving the face, or a large cut on a joint, are best treated by a physician.

W
O
U
N
D
S

Open Wound Care (continued)

IF . . .	THEN . . .
open wound exists	5. Dry the area with a new sterile gauze pad. 6. Use another new sterile pad saturated with rubbing alcohol (isopropyl) on the undamaged skin around the wound. Do *not* put any in the wound since tissue damage can occur. 7. *Optional step*: you can apply some antibiotic skin ointment over the wound (i.e., Polysporin®, Neosporin®, Johnson & Johnson First Aid Cream®, etc.). —Do *not* apply ointment if suture might be needed since it makes suturing more difficult.

W
O
U
N
D
S

Open Wound Care (continued)

IF . . .	THEN . . .
open wound exists	—Do *not* use Mercurochrome, Merthiolate, or iodine since they kill few bacteria, can damage the skin, and some people are allergic to them. Betadine (10%) is an acceptable wound disinfectant, if diluted to 1%.
	8. Place sterile gauze pad over wound and secure it with some sort of gauze roller bandage and adhesive tape.
	—A "nonstickable" dressing works well on abrasions.
	—Use a "band-aid" type of dressing on small cuts.
	—Prevent scabs from breaking open by applying ointment to soften the scab.

W
O
U
N
D
S

Open Wound Care (continued)

If dressing is . . .	THEN . . .
dirty	change it
wet or has been wet	change it
dried, blood-soaked, and bleeding has stopped	change it. When scab or blood sticks to the dressing and the dressing is pulled off roughly, the scab may break and bleeding may restart. If scab sticks to dressing, wet a piece of gauze with 3% hydrogen peroxide, place it on top of the dressing, and let it soak for 1–2 minutes. The hydrogen peroxide will soften the scab and allow removal of the dressing. Keep hydrogen peroxide away from the eyes. Do *not* use warm water since it may soften the tissue and delay healing.

WOUNDS

Open Wound Care (continued)

If dressing is . . .	THEN . . .
covering the wound, but an infection is suspected	change it and look for an infection
not staying in place	change it

W
O
U
N
D
S

Open Wound Care (continued)

IF . . .	THEN . . .
large foreign object is embedded in skin	• do *not* remove or attempt to remove an embedded object • stabilize object in place with bulky dressings and pads • seek medical attention
small foreign object is embedded near the skin's surface and is visible	• use sterile tweezers to pull it out. Tip of a sterile needle can also be used to remove small object • wash area with soap and water • apply a dressing over wound

WOUNDS

Open Wound Care (continued)

IF . . .	THEN . . .
any of these conditions exist: • arterial bleeding • uncontrolled bleeding • deep cuts that: 　—go into the muscle or bone 　—are located on a joint (knee, elbow) 　—tend to gape widely 　—are located on thumb or palm of hand • large or deep puncture wound • dirt and/or debris left in wound • human or animal bite • wound located where scar would be noticeable • eyelid cut • slit lip	• seek medical attention since most may require sutures • try to control bleeding

WOUNDS

Open Wound Care (continued)

If wound has . . .	THEN . . .
• red or discolored skin around it • swelling • warm feeling • pain and tenderness • pus **AND/OR** • athlete feels sick or feverish • athlete has "red streaks" extending up arm or leg from wound	suspect an infection and seek medical attention. • an infection can appear in a wound 2–7 days after injury occurs • infection can be prevented by using soap and water

WOUNDS

Tetanus ("lockjaw") can also occur from an open wound. If the athlete has not had a tetanus shot in the past 5 years, a physician should be consulted. All massive and severe wounds should be seen by a physician and a tetanus shot should be considered.

Bandaging	Open wounds require a dressing and bandage.

Dressings touch the wound and should:
- be sterile. Be careful to touch only the corner of the dressing in order to maintain the dressing's sterility. If a completely sterile dressing is not available, it should be as clean as possible.
- cover entire wound surface. Dressings come in various sizes.
- help control bleeding.

Bandages should:
- be as clean as possible (they do not have to be sterile)
- hold dressings in place
- leave the fingers and toes exposed in order to check changes in blood circulation
- allow the wound to "breathe"
- be snug, but not too tight (complaints of numbness, tingling sensations, or pain indicate a bandage is too tight) or too loose.

The most useful bandage is the self-adhering, form-fitting, gauze roller bandage. This bandage has eliminated the need to know specialized bandaging methods.

Bandage a wound over a joint (elbows, wrists, knees, and ankles) by using the "figure-eight" technique:

1. Go around the limb several times to overlap the dressing's edge.
2. Cross the dressing diagonally.
3. Go around the limb several times.
4. Cross the dressing diagonally, but in the opposite direction as the first diagonal crossing. This makes an "X" over the wound site and forms the figure eight.
5. Repeat the process until the dressing is completely covered and secured.
6. Tape the end of the bandage to prevent unwrapping.

Head and Facial Injuries

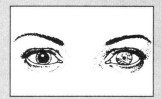

Dangers of Head Injuries

Head injuries can be serious and difficult first aid emergencies to handle. The athlete is often confused or unconscious, making assessment difficult. Many head injuries are life-threatening. If an athlete with a head injury is mishandled, permanent damage or death can occur.

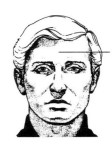

Head
•concussion
•skull
 fracture

Head Injury Care

If head is hit or jarred and the athlete remains CONSCIOUS and . . .	THEN . . .
athlete complains of: • dizziness • ringing in the ears • headache • nausea • blurred vision and any of the following are seen: • blood or clear fluid draining from the ears or nose • bump ("goose egg") or deformity • bleeding • unequal pupils • seizures or convulsions • slurred speech	Proceed as follows: 1. Check for spinal/neck injury by noting arm/leg weakness or paralysis. If little or no reaction occurs when you pinch feet and hands, stabilize head and neck as they were found in order to prevent movement. Tell the athlete not to move. 2. Control bleeding by gently applying direct pressure with a dry, sterile gauze pad. If a skull fracture is suspected, apply pressure around wound edges, not directly on wound.

H
E
A
D

Head Injury Care (continued)

If head is hit or jarred and the athlete remains CONSCIOUS and . . .	THEN . . .
• memory loss • eyes do not track together on an object	3. Applying an ice pack for 20 minutes helps stop any bleeding and reduces pain. 4. Do *not* block any fluid (cerebrospinal fluid and/or blood) coming from an ear. 5. If spinal injury is *not* suspected, keep athlete's upper body elevated—do *not* elevate legs since this increases blood pressure to the brain. Do *not* elevate the athlete's head at the neck since it may obstruct airway. 6. Do *not* give athlete anything to eat or drink. 7. Seek immediate medical attention.

H
E
A
D

Head Injury Care (continued)

If head is hit or jarred and the athlete is UNCONSCIOUS and may have possible . . .	THEN . . .

• breathing difficulty
• blood or clear fluid draining from ears or nose
	proceed as follows:
	1. Assume that a spinal/neck injury exists until proven otherwise.
	2. Check ABCs (airway, breathing, and circulation). Use jaw-thrust method to open airway. Do *not* bend the neck.
	3. Stabilize athlete's head and neck as you found them either by:
	   —using your hands along both sides of the head
	   —placing soft but rigid materials alongside head and neck.

H
E
A
D

- 53 -

Head Injury Care (continued)

If head is hit or jarred and the athlete is UNCONSCIOUS and may have possible . . .	THEN . . .
	4. Control bleeding by gently applying direct pressure with a dry, sterile gauze pad. If skull fracture is suspected, apply pressure around wound edges.
	5. Applying an ice pack for 20 minutes helps stop any bleeding and reduces pain.
	6. If a spinal/neck injury is *not* suspected, try to place athlete in the recovery position (athlete on his/her side, knees bent, bottom arm behind back, top arm's hand under chin).
	7. Seek medical attention.

H
E
A
D

Head Injury Care (continued)

If head is hit or jarred, determine if . . .	THEN . . .
• any loss of consciousness happened. Memory loss, dizziness and ringing in ears may occur without loss of coordination.	Suspect a *mild concussion:* • recovery time will be rapid, but delay return to activity until physician permits
• athlete has been unconscious for 10 seconds to 5 minutes. Accompanied by confusion, moderate dizziness, ringing in ears, unsteadiness, and inability to remember recent events.	Suspect a *moderate concussion:* • avoid vigorous activity for a few days or longer. Resume activity after physician permits.
• athlete has been unconscious for more than 5 minutes. Accompanied by dizziness, ringing in ears, and inability to remember recent events.	Suspect a *severe concussion:* • avoid vigorous activity for a month or longer. Resume activity after neurosurgeon permits.

HEAD

Head Injury Care (continued)

"1–2–3 Rule" for Returning to Activity after a Concussion	
If athlete has . . .	**THEN . . .**
• 1 concussion	athlete is out of the game
• 2 concussions	athlete is out for the season
• 3 concussions	athlete should no longer play
If any of the following signs appear within 48 hours of a head injury . . .	**THEN . . .**
1. **Headache** lasts more than 1–2 days or increases in severity. 2. **Nausea** lasts more than 2 hours. 3. **Vomiting** begins hours after 1–2 episodes have stopped.	**Seek immediate medical attention!**

H
E
A
D

Head Injury Care (continued)

If any of the following signs appear within 48 hours of a head injury . . .	THEN . . .
4. **Athlete cannot answer questions** about recent events (e.g., what day it is, game location, or cannot repeat list of 5–6 numbers). Wake athlete every 2–3 hours to reevaluate memory status by asking questions about recent events or having athlete repeat 5–6 numbers. 5. **Eyes:** • athlete "sees double" • eyes fail to move together • one pupil appears larger than the other	**Seek immediate medical attention!**

H
E
A
D

Head Injury Care (continued)

If any of the following signs appear within 48 hours of a head injury . .	THEN . . .
6. **Muscular paralysis:** athlete has inability to use his/her arms/legs, or is unsteady in walking. 7. **Speech** is slurred or athlete is unable to talk. 8. **Seizures** occur.	**Seek immediate medical attention!**

H
E
A
D

| Warning: | Do *not* attempt to remove a helmet if athlete is unconscious or if spinal injury is suspected. If airway obstruction is suspected or cardiopulmonary resuscitation (CPR) is necessary, remove any face mask with bolt cutters or cut face mask clips with heavy-duty scissors and rotate face mask away. If at all possible, wait for trained emergency medical personnel (i.e., EMTs) to provide care. |

Head Injury Care (continued)

If there is/are . . .	THEN . . .
• pain at injury site • skull deformity (depressions or large swellings known as "goose eggs") • bleeding from ears and/or nose • leakage of clear or pink, watery fluid dripping from nose or ear (known as cerebrospinal fluid) • discoloration under the eyes ("raccoon eyes" or "black eyes") • bruise or discoloration behind an ear (Battle's sign) • unequal pupils • profuse scalp bleeding if skin is broken (scalp wound may expose skull or brain tissue) • nausea and dizziness	1. Give first aid as for an athlete who has sustained either a scalp wound or a brain concussion as described above. 2. Seek immediate medical attention.

HEAD

Jaw Injury

Virtually every jaw injury is the result of a direct blow to the area. In addition to the injured jaw, evaluation for a neck or head injury should be considered.

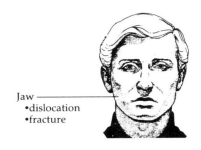

Jaw
•dislocation
•fracture

Jaw Injury Care

IF . . .	THEN . . .
jaw received direct hit and athlete: • cannot close mouth or talk • has numb face • has severe pain • has visible deformity • has swelling	suspect possible *dislocation:* • Apply an ice pack for 20 minutes. • Immobilize the jaw by wrapping face and head. Show athlete how to quickly remove wrapping in case of vomiting. • Seek immediate medical attention.
blow to jaw causes severe pain: • over bone in upper or lower jaw • radiating from injury when area is touched • while opening and closing mouth and/or biting down • with bleeding around teeth	suspect possible *fracture:* • Apply an ice pack to area for 20 minutes. • Reevaluate after application of an ice pack to area. If area is not pain-free, seek medical evaluation before returning to participation. • Seek immediate medical attention.

H
E
A
D

Jaw Injury Care (continued)

If . . .	THEN . . .
athlete is to return to participation	take the following precautions: 1. Be sure area is protected. 2. Make sure no underlying head injury exists, especially if lower jaw was forced upwards. Refer to head injury evaluation in previous section. 3. Make sure no spinal/neck injury exists—check sensations and movements in the hands. 4. When in doubt, athlete should be medically cleared for participation.

H
E
A
D

Nosebleeds

Types of nosebleeds:

- **Anterior** (front of nose). The most common (90%); bleeding occurs out of one nostril.
- **Posterior** (back of nose). Massive bleeding backward into the mouth or down the back of the throat; bleeding starts on one side, then comes out of both nostrils and down the throat; serious and requires medical attention.

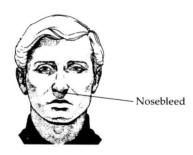

Nosebleed

Nosebleed Care

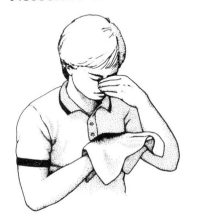

IF . . .	THEN . . .
bleeding appears to be from one nostril (anterior type)	stop bleeding by following these procedures: 1. Reassure and keep him/her quiet. 2. Keep athlete in sitting position. 3. Keep athlete's head tilted slightly forward so that blood can run out the front of the nose, not down the throat. 4. With thumb and finger, apply steady pressure to both nostrils for 5 minutes. Have athlete breathe through his/her mouth.

H
E
A
D

Nosebleed Care (continued)

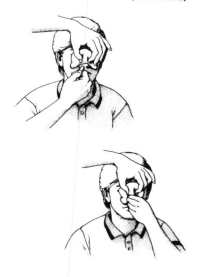

IF ...	THEN ...
	5. Other methods of stopping a nosebleed include: —If bleeding continues, have athlete gently blow nose to remove any clots and excess blood. Press nostrils again for 5 minutes. **OR** —Gently place a cotton ball soaked in water inside nostril. **OR** —Place roll of gauze (the diameter of a pencil in size) between upper lip and teeth/gums and press against it with your fingers. —Apply an ice pack over nose (use along with other methods).

HEAD

Nosebleed Care (continued)

IF . . .	THEN . . .
• bleeding does not stop after second nose pinching attempt	• suspect a posterior nosebleed that requires medical attention
• bleeding happens after a blow to the nose and a broken nose is suspected because of: —swelling —deformity —bleeding coming from both nostrils in large amounts	• suspect a possible fracture • try to stop nosebleed using methods described above • seek medical attention

H
E
A
D

Eye Injuries

The typical eye injury is caused by some form of impact to the eye, cheek, or possibly forehead. Medical evaluation before returning to participation is necessary if there is prolonged blurred or double vision, blood in the colored portion of the eye, or pain. A superficial symptom may indicate a more serious underlying problem. Eye injuries should not be taken lightly; medical assessment is recommended for any painful eye injury.

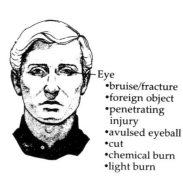

Eye
- bruise/fracture
- foreign object
- penetrating injury
- avulsed eyeball
- cut
- chemical burn
- light burn

Eye Injury Care

IF . . .	THEN . . .
blow to eye and/or surrounding area happens and . . . • swelling and discoloration is seen • severe pain occurs • there are accompanying cuts, bleeding, and bruise marks	suspect *bruise* and/or *fracture*: 1. Apply an ice pack for 20–30 minutes if no damage to eyeball exists. Athlete can remove it periodically for comfort. Do **not** apply pressure on the eye. 2. Place dry cloth or 3–4 sterile gauze pads between ice pack and eye. 3. Seek medical attention for: —blurred and/or double vision (avoid blowing nose until medically examined) —sensation lost above the eyebrow or over the cheek (nerve damage) —"black eye."

H
E
A
D

Eye Injury Care (continued)

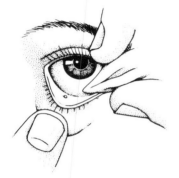

IF . . .	THEN . . .
	4. Keep athlete in sitting position. 5. If head and neck injuries also exist, do *not* move the head; wait for the EMS system.
eye has "foreign object or debris" sensation, blurred vision, redness, or painful and excessive watering	suspect *foreign object* or *debris in eye:* 1. Do not rub. 2. Lift athlete's upper eyelid over the lower eyelid. Have athlete blink a few times. 3. Rinse eye gently with warm water. Help hold eye open. Have athlete look down. Do not rinse if eyeball has cut or puncture wound.

H
E
A
D

Eye Injury Care (continued)

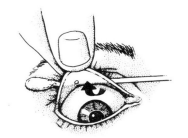

IF . . .	THEN . . .
	4. Examine lower eyelid by pulling it down gently. If object seen, flush the eye with water. Examine upper eyelid by grasping lashes of upper eyelid; place a swab across upper eyelid and roll eyelid upward over the swab. If object is seen, remove it with a moistened sterile gauze pad. Have athlete look down.
	5. If object remains, patch both eyes and seek medical attention.

H
E
A
D

Eye Injury Care (continued)

IF . . .	THEN . . .
object is impaled or embedded	suspect *penetrating injury:* 1. Do *not* remove foreign objects impaled or stuck in the eye. 2. Stabilize object and protect eye by: —placing a roll of gauze on each side of the object —placing paper cup or cardboard cone over eye. 3. Cover undamaged eye with a patch in order to stop movement of damaged eye. 4. Seek medical attention.

H
E
A
D

Eye Injury Care (continued)

IF . . .	THEN . . .
blood appears in eye area	suspect a *cut eye* and/or *cut eyelid:* 1. Bandage both eyes lightly and seek immediate medical attention. 2. Do *not* attempt to wash out the eye or remove an object stuck in the eye. 3. Do *not* apply hard pressure to injured eye or eyelid.
chemical gets into eye	suspect a *chemical burn:* 1. Flood eye with warm water **immediately** for 15–20 minutes. You can't use too much water. 2. Use your fingers to keep eye open as wide as possible. 3. Have athlete roll eyeball as much as possible. 4. Do *not* use eye cup.

H
E
A
D

Eye Injury Care (continued)

IF . . .	THEN . . .
eye feels scratchy and painful 1–6 hours after exposure to snow or sun	suspect *light burn* ("*snowblindness*"): 1. Cover both eyes with cold, moist compresses. 2. Keep athlete resting in dark room. 3. Seek medical attention.

H
E
A
D

Ear Injuries

Impact or a direct blow to the ear can cause a bruise to the outer ear or damage to the inner ear. An injury may include damage to the ear drum, which requires prompt medical attention. Also, any fluid coming from the inner ear requires immediate medical attention. It is not uncommon in head injuries for the ears to have a "ringing" sensation.

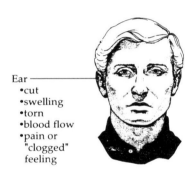

Ear
•cut
•swelling
•torn
•blood flow
•pain or "clogged" feeling

Ear Injury Care

If external ear . . .	THEN . . .
is scratched or cut	• clean wound • apply gauze dressing and bandage
receives a blow, or rubbing of outer ear causes swelling of outer ear tissue	• apply ice pack held by an elastic bandage • athlete can remove as needed for comfort • seek medical attention if swelling continues after this treatment in order to prevent "cauliflower ear"
is torn or avulsed	• place torn part back into normal position • apply bulky dressing over top of ear and several gauze pads behind ear • bandage with self-adhering roller bandage

HEAD

Ear Injury Care (continued)

If internal ear has . . .	THEN . . .
flow of blood from ear canal or accumulation of blood in ear canal	• do *not* pack ear canal with cotton or gauze • apply gauze pad over external ear • seek medical attention
loss of hearing, "clogged ear" feeling, or ear pain	• do *not* allow athlete to hit or thump head to try to restore hearing • check for clear or bloody fluids in ear • treat for possible head injury • seek medical attention

H
E
A
D

Dental Injuries

Many teeth that could have been saved were lost because of improper care at the injury scene. The introduction of the mouth guard in the 1950s has almost eliminated loss of teeth and sharply reduced mouth injuries. The mouth guard is now required safety equipment in contact/collision sports, such as football, and becoming more popular in other high impact sports. Protective face masks are effective in preventing dental injuries and are required in several sports.

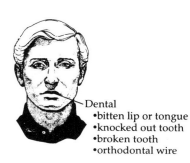

Dental
•bitten lip or tongue
•knocked out tooth
•broken tooth
•orthodontal wire

Dental Injury Care

IF . . .	THEN . . .
lip or tongue bleeds	suspect *bitten lip* or *tongue:* 1. Apply pressure to bleeding area with sterile gauze. 2. If lip is swollen, apply an ice pack. 3. Seek medical attention if bleeding continues or for severe wound.
tooth is knocked out and socket is painful and bleeding	follow these procedures: 1. Find tooth and gently rinse it in running water. 2. Do *not* put tooth in alcohol or scrub it. Do *not* touch the tooth's roots. 3. Place tooth in cup of cold whole milk if available. Do *not* use low-fat or powdered milk or milk by-products (e.g., yogurt).

H
E
A
D

Dental Injury Care (continued)

IF . . .	THEN . . .
	4. Take victim and tooth to dentist immediately (within 30 minutes).
	5. The tooth could be placed in victim's mouth to keep it moist, but it may be swallowed.
	6. Control bleeding from socket with gauze pad.
	7. A partly extracted tooth can be pushed back into place without rinsing the tooth. Seek a dentist so that the loose tooth can be stabilized.

H
E
A
D

Dental Injury Care (continued)

IF . . .	THEN . . .
	8. If dentist is not nearby (farther than 30 minutes away), replant tooth by first running cool water over it to clean away debris (do not scrub); then gently reposition it into the socket, using adjacent teeth as a guide. See a dentist as soon as possible.
tooth is broken and is painful and sensitive to heat and cold	take these precautions: 1. Clean any dirt, blood, and debris from injured area with sterile gauze pad or clean cloth and warm water. 2. Apply an ice pack on the face next to injured tooth. 3. If jaw fracture is suspected, stabilize jaw with bandage under the chin. 4. Seek a dentist immediately.

HEAD

Dental Injury Care (continued)

IF . . .	THEN . . .
orthodontal wire or appliance causes: • irritation **OR** • becomes loose **OR** • wire embeds in cheek, tongue, or gum tissue	proceed as follows: 1. cover end of wire with small cotton ball or piece of gauze, until it can be seen by dentist. 2. Take appliance and the piece and see dentist. 3. Do *not* try to remove it. See dentist immediately.

H
E
A
D

CHAPTER

6

Neck and Shoulder Injuries

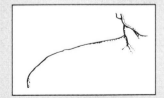

Neck Injury

Neck
- fracture
- sprain
- contusion
- strain

Impact to the neck will routinely cause a strain or sprain. These injuries can cause pain in the neck itself or pain to shoot down an arm to the hand. A neck fracture can be life-threatening or cause paralysis. Emergency care is absolutely necessary for a catastrophic injury. Medical evaluation is strongly recommended for sprains, contusions, and strains prior to a return to participation.

Neck Injury Care

IF . . .	THEN . . .

athlete received a blow causing head to come forward into chest or snap backwards and if:
• *unconscious:*
  1. Test responses by pinching the athlete's hands (either palms or back) and feet (soles or tops of bare feet). No reaction could mean spinal cord damage.
  2. Assume a spinal injury exists.
	suspect possible *neck fracture* or *other catastrophic injury:*
	1. Check and monitor the ABCs (airway, breathing, and circulation) if athlete is motionless and/or unconscious. See page 21 for proper techniques.
	2. Call and wait for the EMS system because of their training and equipment.

Neck Injury Care (continued)

IF . . .	THEN . . .

• *conscious*
AND:
• has a head injury
• complains about his/her hands "burning"
• has numbness, tingling, weakness, or burning in arms and/or legs
THEN ask athlete:
   —Is there pain?
   —Can you move your fingers?
   —Can you move your toes?
	3. Stabilize athlete against any movement. Do this by holding the head still. For conscious athlete, tell him/her not to move.
	4. Treat for shock by keeping athlete warm.
	
	Improper care could cause a lifetime of paralysis.

N
E
C
K

Neck Injury Care (continued)

IF . . .	THEN . . .
athlete comes from participation under own power, but: • complains of burning and tingling from the neck, down the arm, and toward the hand • has pain and weakness with neck motions—up and down, and right to left • has pain and weakness with arm motions • has weakness with grip strength	suspect *severe sprain* or *contusion* with *possible nerve injury* (known as a *"burner"* or *"stinger"*): 1. Stabilize head and spine. 2. Apply an ice pack to area for 30 minutes. 3. Reevaluate after application of ice pack. Seek medical evaluation if pain and weakness are evident. Do not allow athlete to return to participation. 4. Apply an ice pack 3–4 times daily for first 48 hours. 5. Seek medical attention if any weakness is evident.

Neck Injury Care (continued)

IF . . .	THEN . . .
neck has been forced sideways, forward, or backwards **OR** neck was hit directly and: • no burning or tingling is evident as described above • pain with neck motions is mild • weakness and pain with arm motions are mild	suspect *mild strain* or *contusion:* 1. Apply an ice pack to area for 30 minutes. 2. Reevaluate after application of ice pack. If pain and weakness are evident, do not allow athlete to return to participation. 3. Seek medical evaluation if any weakness is evident 48 hours after the injury for appropriate rehabilitation procedures.

N
E
C
K

Shoulder Injuries

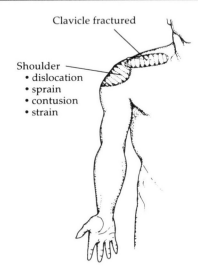

Clavicle fractured

Shoulder
• dislocation
• sprain
• contusion
• strain

Shoulder injuries can range from mild to ones that pose medical emergencies. A dislocated shoulder, which usually occurs during contact sports, requires immediate medical attention. Typically, sprains and contusions will not be emergencies, but can produce pain and cause an athlete to miss from a few days to several weeks of participation. Strains associated with throwing injuries can also have a wide range of severity and can occur instantly or gradually over time. A shoulder dislocation can be confused with a shoulder separation. The key difference is that in separation, the shoulder joint and upper arm remain mobile. In dislocation, the mobility is lost.

Shoulder Injury Care

If athlete . . .	THEN . . .
• fell on his/her shoulder • had arm rotated or twisted • has history of shoulder dislocations **AND** if athlete has: • severe pain at front of shoulder • visible deformity • been holding the injured arm with the uninjured arm slightly away from the chest • swelling • bruising • tenderness • dent or hollow place in the deltoid muscle	suspect a *shoulder dislocation:* 1. Do *not* try to force, twist, or pull the shoulder back in place because it may cause nerve or blood vessel injury. 2. Place rolled towels, rolled blanket, or pillow between upper arm and chest. 3. If athlete is sitting, apply an arm sling and swathe (binder). 4. Use a Sam® Splint to form a triangular "airplane" splint between upper arm and chest. (See Appendix B.) 5. Apply an ice pack to the area for 15 minutes, if it can be tolerated. 6. Seek immediate medical attention. *Improper care of a shoulder dislocation can cause more severe damage than the initial injury produced.*

N
E
C
K

Shoulder Injury Care (continued)

If athlete . . .	THEN . . .
• fell on outstretched arm • received a direct blow to the clavicle (collarbone) or shoulder **AND** if athlete has: • severe pain over injured area • been holding the injured arm against the chest with the uninjured arm • not moved the arm because of pain • swelling • visible deformity • tenderness • "dropped" shoulder • bruising	suspect a *fractured clavicle (collarbone):* 1. Treat for shock by keeping athlete warm and elevating the legs 8–12 inches in a straight position. If athlete has head injury or difficulty breathing normally, do ***not*** elevate feet, but elevate shoulders. 2. Place arm in a sling and swathe (binder). 3. Apply an ice pack to the area for 30 minutes, 3–4 times during the next 24 hours. 4. Seek immediate medical attention.

Shoulder Injury Care (continued)

IF . . .	THEN . . .
injury resulted from: • shoulder being hit directly on the tip • arm being forced sideways, backwards, or downwards • athlete falling on outstretched hand with elbow straight • athlete falling on elbow with upper arm straight • sudden throwing force **AND** • athlete felt "pop" sensation at the time of injury • shoulder is tender to touch and appears unusually elevated • pain and weakness are experienced when athlete moves shoulder forward, sideways, or backwards • athlete has severe pain • a visible deformity exists • swelling occurs	suspect *shoulder sprain, contusion,* or *strain:* 1. Place arm in sling and swathe (binder). 2. Apply an ice pack to area for 30 minutes, 3–4 times during the first 24 hours. 3. Wrap with a 6-inch elastic bandage. 4. Seek medical attention before allowing the athlete to return to participation.

N
E
C
K

IF . . .	THEN . . .
cause of injury is same as above **AND** • athlete is able to move shoulder forward, sideways, backwards, and in a circular rotation with minimal soreness • no pain occurs when gentle pressure is applied to tip of shoulder	suspect *mild sprain, contusion,* or *strain:* 1. Apply an ice pack to the area for 30 minutes, 3–4 times during the first 24 hours. 2. Reevaluate range of motion and tenderness after application of ice pack. 3. Return to participation is possible if: —pain at injury site is tolerable —no pain results when moving shoulder forward, sideways, backwards, and in a circular rotation —all range of motion is pain-free against mild resistance—and similar in strength to healthy arm —simulated sports activities are painless on bench or sidelines —area can be padded for protection as needed.

Shoulder Injury Care (continued)

IF . . .	THEN . . .
	4. Apply an ice pack 3–4 times during first 24 hours..
	5. If pain increases in the first 24 hours, make athlete cease participation and seek medical examination before allowing athlete to return to participation.

Torso
Injuries

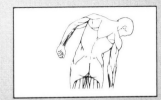

Chest, Rib, and Mid-Back Injuries

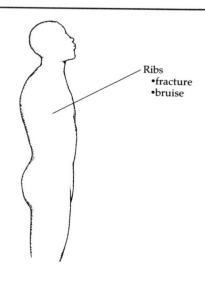

Ribs
•fracture
•bruise

These injuries can be very painful, and are generally caused by a blow to the area or a torsion strain. On rare occasions, internal organs can be damaged by the injury. Significant pain can be associated with a lung injury. Bloody urine can be from kidney trauma.

Chest, Rib, and Mid-Back Injury Care

IF . . .	THEN . . .
direct hit produces: • pain over area • tenderness to touch **And if:** • squeezing the rib cage causes pain over the injury site (known as the "rib spring" technique) • breathing or coughing produces sharp pain • trunk rotation is painful	suspect *rib fracture* or *deep bruise:* 1. Apply an ice pack for 30 minutes. 2. Splint area with compression wrap comfortably applied around chest **OR** have victim hold a pillow or other soft, bulky object against injured area. 3. Medical evaluation needed if pain is over bony area or if breathing is painful with shortness of breath. 4. If *not* fractured, allow athlete to return to participation if breathing is pain-free and area is well padded.

T
O
R
S
O

Chest, Rib, and Mid-Back Injury Care (continued)

IF . . .	THEN . . .
excessive torsion produces: • pop or pulling sensation within muscular soft tissue • tenderness and soreness to touch • ache with trunk twist or other motion • soreness with deep breathing	suspect *muscle strain (tear)*: 1. Apply an ice pack for 30 minutes, 3–4 times daily during first 48 hours. 2. Maintain pain-free flexibility. Do *not* force flexibility. 3. Return to participation if area is adequately padded and flexibility is pain-free.

T
O
R
S
O

Back Injuries

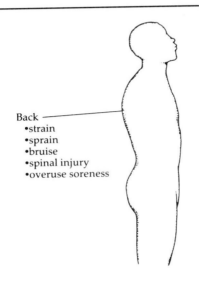

Back
- strain
- sprain
- bruise
- spinal injury
- overuse soreness

Low and mid-back injuries generally result from a direct trauma, such as a tackle, or indirectly, such as a torsion strain from throwing. Vertebrae, the bones of the spine, can be fractured like any other bone in the body. This fracture is severe because it can damage the spinal cord. Muscular strains and contusions can also be painful and limit the athlete's flexibility. As with chest injuries, a low back injury may also cause trauma to a kidney, and blood in the urine requires prompt medical attention.

Back Injury Care

If athlete has . . .	THEN . . .
• head injury (about 15–20% of athletes with head injuries also have neck and spinal cord injuries) in which the head was snapped suddenly • painful movement of arms and/or legs • numbness, tingling, weakness, or burning sensation in arms or legs • paralysis of arms and/or legs • deformity or odd-looking angle of athlete's head and neck • tenderness over any point of neck or spine	suspect *spinal cord damage*. **Proceed with caution!** 1. Check and monitor the ABCs (airway, breathing, and circulation) and treat accordingly. Do *not* use head-tilt method because it would move the neck—jut jaw forward instead. Keep head and neck still. 2. Call the emergency medical services (EMS) system because of their training and equipment to handle an athlete with possible spinal cord damage.

T
O
R
S
O

If athlete has . . .	THEN . . .
Ask the conscious athlete the following questions: —Is there pain? —Can you move your feet? Ask athlete to move his/her foot against your hand. ' —Can you move your fingers? Movement indicates nerve pathways are intact. Ask athlete to grip your hand. For an unconscious athlete: —Test responses by pinching athlete's hands (either palms or backs of hands) and soles or tops of bare feet. No reaction could mean spinal cord damage. —If not sure about a possible spinal injury, assume that the athlete has one until proven otherwise.	3. Stabilize athlete against any movement. Do *not* move the neck to reposition it except when danger is present. Bring help to the athlete, *not* the reverse. 4. Tell the conscious athlete *not* to move. Place objects on both sides of the head to prevent it from rolling from side to side.

T
O
R
S
O

Back Injury Care (continued)

If athlete has . . .	THEN . . .
an injury that is the result of direct hit or excessive twist producing: • tenderness to touch • pain at injury site • stiffness and pain with motions • pain radiating toward hip or down one leg **And later:** • extreme pain when urinating • blood in urine	suspect *deep bruise, kidney bruise,* or *significant strain* or *sprain* 1. Treat with an ice pack for 20–30 minutes at the time of injury and 3–4 times through the first 48 hours. 2. Encourage pain-free flexibility. Do *not* force stretching. 3. Do *not* allow athlete to return to participation if flexibility is incomplete or painful. 4. Wake athlete during the night of the original injury in order to gently stretch and apply an ice pack. 5. Seek medical attention if there is no reduction of pain within 48 hours **OR** if there is a tingling or numbness running down one or both legs. 6. Seek medical attention if blood in the urine appears.

T
O
R
S
O

Back Injury Care (continued)

If athlete has . . .	THEN . . .
an ongoing ache **AND:** • motion produces pain (e.g., tennis serve) • pain increases with activity • pain subsides when activity stops	suspect *overuse soreness:* 1. Heat area for 20 minutes and stretch well prior to activity. 2. Wrap or brace for support and heat retention. 3. Apply an ice pack for 30 minutes after activity. 4. Seek medical attention for rehabilitation program.

Seek medical attention for any back problem that:
- hurts so much that the athlete can't sleep
- after a few days still hurts
- has any one of these symptoms:
  —pain that radiates to other parts of the body
  —numbness or tingling in arms or legs
  —sudden weakness in arms or legs.

T
O
R
S
O

Abdominal Injury

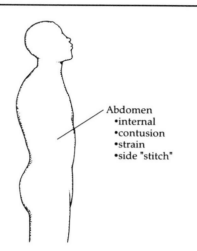

Abdomen
•internal
•contusion
•strain
•side "stitch"

Abdominal injuries are usually caused by blows to the stomach or solar plexus—a network of nerves located behind the stomach—causing the diaphragm to spasm. The most serious abdominal injuries are those that damage internal organs, particularly the spleen and kidney. Any of these can be a frightening experience for the athlete. The athlete should not return to participation until there is no pain. If internal damage is suspected, seek medical attention immediately, regardless if it is at the time of injury or several hours later.

Abdominal Injury Care

IF . . .	THEN . . .
injury is from a direct hit to the abdomen producing: • pain or tenderness in the abdomen • stiffness or soreness • guarding of the abdomen • legs drawn up to the chest • nausea **And** hours later there is: • pain in the shoulder on the same side as the injury • nausea and/or vomiting • blood in the urine	suspect possible *internal abdominal damage:* 1. Place athlete on his/her back with legs flexed at the knees. 2. Hold a pillow or other soft, bulky object against abdomen. 3. Delayed shoulder pain may indicate internal damage. Seek immediate medical attention. 4. Apply an ice pack for 30 minutes over the site. 5. Return to participation should not occur if flexibility is painful.

T
O
R
S
O

Abdominal Injury Care (continued)

IF . . .	THEN . . .
injury from a direct hit to the abdomen producing: • loss of breath ("wind knocked out")—cannot breathe in or exhale • mild abdominal pain AND . . . • if athlete starts hyperventilating	suspect *mild contusion:* 1. Place athlete in a comfortable position, usually lying on his/her back with legs flexed. 2. Loosen any tight clothing and encourage athlete to take short breaths in through the nose and long breaths out through the mouth. 3. Do *not* lift athlete by the belt in an attempt to help his/her breathing. 4. Refer to evaluation for possible internal abdominal damage above.

Abdominal Injury Care (continued)

IF . . .	THEN . . .
	5. Do *not* use the old method of treating hyperventilation (breathing into a paper bag) because it places stress on the heart and respiratory system. Breathing into a bag rarely restores blood-gas balance. The athlete may be having a heart attack, breathing difficulty, or another health problem. Instead, have the athlete breathe slowly.

TORSO

Abdominal Injury Care (continued)

IF . . .	THEN . . .
trunk is twisted producing: • soreness with forward/ backward motions • pain and tenderness to the touch • ache with deep breathing/ coughing	suspect *muscle strain (tear)*: 1. Apply an ice pack for 30 minutes, 3–4 times daily. 2. Maintain pain-free flexibility. Do *not* force flexibility.
a cramping pain happens during running	suspect a *"stitch" in side:* 1. Raise arm on affected side overhead as high as possible. **AND/OR** 2. Bend forward at the waist. 3. If pain continues seek medical attention.

T
O
R
S
O

Hip and Buttocks Injuries

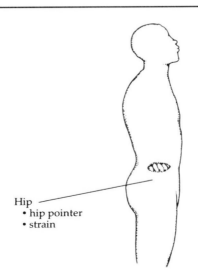

Hip
• hip pointer
• strain

The "hip pointer" injury is often quite painful, to a point that the athlete thinks the bone has been fractured. This injury can affect general trunk motions such as bending and walking, or breathing. Standard care for a "hip pointer" is beneficial, but the injury does require a thorough medical examination. Hip muscle strains can occur from excessive torsion while running.

Hip and Buttocks Injury Care

If athlete . . .	THEN . . .
receives direct hit producing: • immediate pain • tenderness to the touch • swelling **AND** later: • has pain and difficulty bending trunk forward, backward, or sideways • is unable to run • has pain with deep breathing, coughing, sneezing • cannot move thigh forward	suspect *"hip pointer"* or *contused buttocks:* 1. Apply wet 4-inch or 6-inch double-length elastic wrap for compression. 2. Apply an ice pack to area for 20–30 minutes. 3. Have athlete stretch in order to maintain pain-free flexibility. Do not force flexibility. 4. Wake athlete during the first night of injury to walk and gently stretch. 5. Do *not* allow athlete to return to participation while flexibility or sports movements are painful. Seek medical attention if pain increases or does not improve within 48 hours.

TORSO

Hip and Buttocks Injury Care (continued)

If athlete . . .	THEN . . .
	6. Continue ice pack applications 30 minutes, 3–4 times daily for first 48 hours. Do not apply heat.
while running feels: • pop or pulling from buttocks or side of hip **AND,** at the time of injury has: • tenderness to the touch • sense of firmness when area is pressed • soreness while moving leg up and down, or sideways	suspect *muscle strain:* 1. Apply an ice pack for 20–30 minutes at the time of injury and 3–4 times daily for first 48 hours. 2. Follow Step #s 3, 4, and 5 above.

Hip and Buttocks Injury Care (continued)

If athlete . . .	THEN . . .
has no pain running at normal speed without a limp: • forward/backward • sideways and changing direction • in figure eights	1. Allow athlete to return to participation 2. Apply an ice pack after activity.

T
O
R
S
O

Groin Injuries

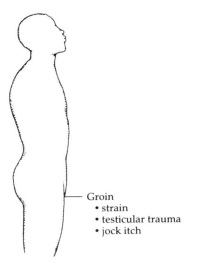

Groin
• strain
• testicular trauma
• jock itch

Groin strains are caused by sudden and quick change of direction or by twisting the thigh while the legs are spread apart. Much like hamstring and thigh strains, a groin strain can occur early in the season or if the athlete is not adequately warmed up or stretched.

Groin Injury Care

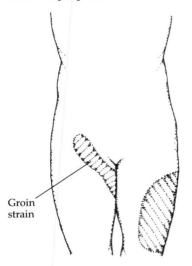

Groin
strain

If athlete has . . .	THEN . . .
felt a pop or tearing while running that produces: • pain and tenderness • soreness when moving leg sideways • swelling • firmness of site when pressed	suspect a *muscle strain with possible tear* (*significant strain*): 1. Wrap compression bandage with pad over area. 2. Apply an ice pack with compression for 20–30 minutes, 3–4 times daily during first 48 hours. 3. Have athlete maintain as much pain-free flexibility as possible. Do *not* force stretching. 4. Wake athlete during the first night to gently stretch area.

Groin Injury Care (continued)

If athlete has . . .	THEN . . .
muscle stretch without a pop or tearing and has: • minimal or no pain when area is pressed or probed • no swelling or abnormal firmness when area is pressed • normal flexibility **AND** can run at normal speed painlessly without a limp: • straight forward and backward • in figure eights • cutting and changing direction	suspect a *muscle stretch without a tear* (*mild strain*): 1. Apply an ice pack for 20–30 minutes, 3–4 times daily during first 48 hours. 2. Have athlete try to achieve as much pain-free flexibility as possible. Do *not* force stretching. 3. If running is pain-free, wrap or brace the muscle in order for athlete to return to participation.

TORSO

Groin Injury Care (continued)

IF . . .	THEN . . .
injury is from a direct hit to the testicles producing: • loss of breath • local sharp pain • immediate cramping causing athlete to "double up" with pain	suspect *mild testicular trauma:* 1. Place athlete into a crouch position, much like a baseball catcher. 2. Have athlete bounce up and down until relieved of pain. 3. If Step #2 is not effective, have athlete sit up with legs extended on the ground or floor. Lift him up from under the arms about 6–8 inches and drop him. This step can be repeated 2–3 times. This procedure usually eliminates the spasm and provides instant relief from pain and discomfort.

Groin Injury Care (continued)

IF . . .	THEN . . .
	4. Another method is to have the athlete lie on his back. Push his thighs up to his chest, keeping his knees about 15 inches apart.
	5. Another method involves applying ice packs to help prevent swelling and reduce pain.
	6. Seek medical attention if swelling, continued dull pain, sudden pain, nausea, or vomiting occur.
injury is ongoing and getting worse with time **AND** • pain occurs with sports activity • gradual weakness happens with sports activity	suspect *overuse strain:* 1. Apply an ice pack to the area after completing sports activity. 2. Apply heat and have athlete do a thorough stretching and warm-up routine before activity.

T
O
R
S
O

Groin Injury Care (continued)

IF . . .	THEN . . .
	3. Seek medical evaluation and rehabilitation program.
genital area has: • burning pain • itching • rash (scrotum usually not affected)	suspect *jock itch:* 1. Tell athlete to keep area dry (e.g., by changing wet, sweaty clothing and using powder to absorb sweat). 2. Have athlete apply antifungal cream (e.g., Tinactin™, Micatin™) 3 times daily.

T
O
R
S
O

Injuries to the
Upper Extremities

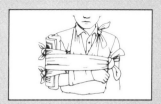

Upper Arm Injuries

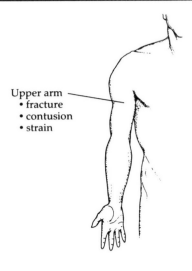

Upper arm
• fracture
• contusion
• strain

Although a fracture of the humerus is rare, complications may happen in upper arm injuries because of the closeness of nerves and blood vessels to the bone. One by-product of an upper arm injury is a "calcium deposit" that can develop at the site of direct trauma. This deposit grows over time and can limit normal muscle function and athletic skill.

Upper Arm Injury Care

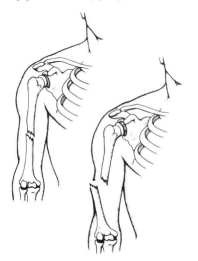

IF . . .	THEN . . .
athlete received a: • direct blow • twist or fall on the outstretched arm **AND** any one or any combination of these occur: • Severe pain • Swelling • Visible deformity • Tender if touched	suspect possible *fracture:* • *Closed fracture*—overlaying skin has not been damaged. • *Open fracture*—overlaying skin has been damaged. The bone may not always be seen in the wound. 1. Treat for shock by keeping athlete warm and elevating straight legs 8–12 inches. 2. Do *not* move arm. 3. Apply an ice pack for 20–30 minutes.

U
P
P
E
R

Upper Arm Injury Care (continued)

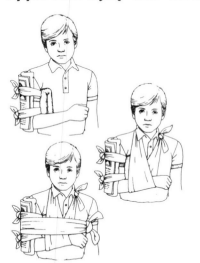

IF . . .	THEN . . .
	4. Immobilize arm by one of several methods: —Rigid splint: apply board or Sam® Splint (see Appendix B) to include joints above and below the fracture site. Place towel or other cushioning between arm and chest and apply arm sling and swathe (binder). —Soft splint: apply arm sling and swathe (binder) with a towel or other cushioning between arm and chest. 5. Seek immediate medical attention.

U
P
P
E
R

IF . . .	THEN . . .
arm was hit and has: • swelling over area • pain over area • bruise beginning (first redness, later turning to "black and blue")	suspect a *contusion* (bruise): 1. Apply an ice pack for 30 minutes, 3–4 times during first 24 hours. 2. Apply elastic wrap.
muscle feels like it's in a spasm and pain occurs when moving or stretching	suspect a *strain:* 1. Apply an ice pack for 30 minutes. 2. Apply elastic wrap.

U
P
P
E
R

Elbow Injuries

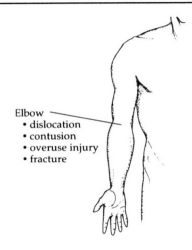

Elbow
• dislocation
• contusion
• overuse injury
• fracture

More often than not, elbow injuries are nagging nuisances; occasionally an elbow will be sprained or become strained. Rarely will an elbow dislocate; however, when this occurs it is a significant medical emergency requiring immediate care. Elbow contusions can be serious because of possible nerve injury.

Elbow Injury Care

IF . . .	THEN . . .
athlete has: • visible elbow deformity • severe pain • displacement of the upper arm forward toward the wrist • "locked" elbow • numbness or paralysis below the injured elbow • swelling • bruising	suspect *dislocated elbow*. 1. Do *not* try moving or forcing elbow joint back into its normal position. 2. Apply an ice pack to the area if athlete can tolerate it. 3. Place arm into a sling, but keep elbow in the position found—do *not* move it. 4. Seek immediate medical attention. *Improper care of an elbow dislocation can result in more severe damage (to nerves and/or blood vessels) than initially produced.*

Elbow Injury Care (continued)

IF . . .	THEN . . .
athlete's elbow was hit directly and he/she has: • burning or tingling sensation running from the elbow toward (and/maybe including) the fingers • weakness and soreness when bending and straightening the elbow • weakness while moving hand, including making a fist and gripping	suspect *nerve contusion:* 1. Apply an ice pack to the area for 30 minutes. 2. After the application of the ice pack, compare motion and strength of the injured elbow with that of the healthy elbow. 3. Do *not* allow athlete to return to participation if tingling and/or weakness are evident. 4. Seek medical evaluation if tingling and/or weakness continue for 24 hours. 5. Apply an ice pack for 30 minutes, 3–4 times daily for first 48 hours.

U
P
P
E
R

Elbow Injury Care (continued)

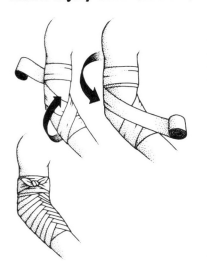

IF . . .	THEN . . .
athlete has been hit on back of elbow or has landed directly on tip of elbow or outstretched hand **AND** has: • tenderness at tip of elbow • soreness with straightening and bending • puffiness at tip of elbow **OR** • "pop" sensation at time of injury • pain and apprehension while fully straightening elbow alone • weakness with fully straightened elbow	suspect *joint contusion* or *sprain*: 1. Apply an ice pack to area for 30 minutes. 2. Apply elastic wrap over elbow. 3. Reevaluate tenderness, motion, and strength as noted above. 4. Allow athlete to return to participation if: —pain is tolerable —motion is painless —simulated sports actions are painless (while on bench or sidelines) —area is padded as needed (or taped) —no numbness or weakness exists from elbow to fingers. 5. Apply an ice pack for 30 minutes, 3–4 times daily for first 48 hours.

U
P
P
E
R

Elbow Injury Care (continued)

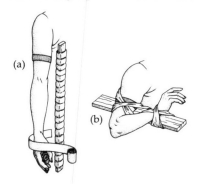

(a)

(b)

IF . . .	THEN . . .
repetitive action produces ongoing pain and: • pain increases while using arm • causes gradual grip weakness • elbow fatigues quicker than normal	suspect an *overuse injury* (*"tennis" elbow* or *"little league" elbow*): 1. Apply heat before activity; have athlete wear brace or rubber sleeve on elbow. 2. Apply an ice pack for 30 minutes after completion of activity. 3. Seek medical evaluation for appropriate rehabilitation program.
after a direct blow or fall on outstretched hand, athlete has: • severe pain • swelling • possible visible deformity • numbness or coldness below elbow	suspect a *fracture:* 4. Do ***not*** move elbow. 5. Splint elbow in the position found in order to prevent nerve and blood vessel damage: —If straight, keep splinted elbow straight. —If bent, keep elbow bent. 6. Seek immediate medical attention.

UPPER

Forearm and Wrist Injuries

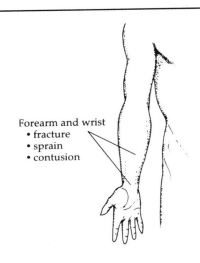

Forearm and wrist
- fracture
- sprain
- contusion

Forearm injuries usually result from a direct blow; wrist injuries can occur in the same way or by falling on an outstretched hand. Fractures to the large forearm bones can be obvious, while some fractures of the small bones in the wrist can be very subtle. Wrist sprains are common in many sports and a return to participation is based on pain and functional ability.

Forearm and Wrist Injury Care

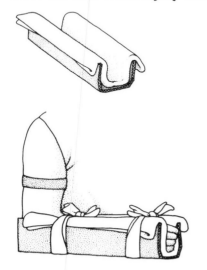

IF . . .	THEN . . .
athlete has pain in the forearm or wrist from: • direct blow • falling on outstretched hand **AND** has • visible deformity • severe pain radiating up and down from the injury site • inability to move wrist or pain while moving wrist **OR** • wrist is painful on thumb side and pain continues into next day	suspect possible *fracture:* 1. Treat for shock by keeping athlete warm and lying down with straight legs elevated 8–12 inches. 2. Apply an ice pack to area for 30 minutes. 3. Apply a splint from tip of elbow to fingers. (See Appendix B for instructions on how to apply a Sam® Splint to the forearm.) If possible, position hand in a thumb-up position. 4. Seek medical attention and later an evaluation prior to athlete's returning to participation.

U
P
P
E
R

Forearm and Wrist Injury Care (continued)

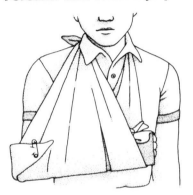

IF . . .	THEN . . .
injury is caused by landing on wrist or outstretched hand **AND** • pain at injury site does not radiate away from site • wrist motions are with little pain • swelling occurs • bruise appears (begins with redness and progresses to "black and blue")	suspect *sprain* or *contusion:* 1. Apply an ice pack to area for 30 minutes. 2. Reevaluate motion after completion of ice pack application. If motions are painful and limited, seek medical evaluation prior to athlete's return to participation. 3. If motion is tolerable, athlete's return to participation is possible with supportive taping or padding. 4. If area is swollen and motion is painful and/or limited 24 hours after initial injury, seek medical attention.

U
P
P
E
R

Forearm and Wrist Injury Care (continued)

IF . . .	THEN . . .
athlete returns to participation, the following must be accomplished: • movement is pain-free • grip strength of injured forearm or wrist is comparable to healthy one • functional needs (i.e., grasping tennis racquet or throwing) are essentially pain-free	for athlete to return to participation: 1. Support injury with appropriate taping or padding as needed. 2. Apply an ice pack after daily participation as long as soreness persists.
ongoing pain is at the base of the thumb in the wrist and: • injury seems like a sprain that is slow to heal • there is some soreness with wrist movements • there is some weakness with wrist movements	suspect possible *fracture:* 1. Seek medical evaluation prior to athlete's return to participation.

U
P
P
E
R

Finger Injuries

Finger
- fracture
- dislocation
- contusion
- sprain
- blood clot under nail

Finger injuries occur in every sport. Most are not severe, but in rare instances a finger can dislocate—producing a grotesque abnormality which requires immediate medical attention. Fractures, sprains, and contusions often resemble each other and can be evaluated using similar methods.

Finger Injury Care

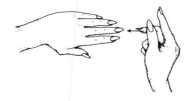

IF . . .	THEN . . .

finger or thumb has:
• visible deformity
• pain
• numbness
• swelling
• tenderness to touch
	suspect a possible *fracture* and/or *dislocation:*
	1. Test for a finger fracture:
	   —If possible, straighten the fingers and place them on a hard surface.
	   —Tap the tip of the injured finger toward the hand. Pain lower down in the finger or into the hand can indicate a fracture.
	2. Do ***not*** try to realign a dislocation.
	3. Gently apply an ice pack.

U
P
P
E
R

Finger Injury Care (continued)

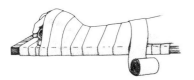

IF . . .	THEN . . .
	4. Splint the finger by either: —"buddy" taping for support. For a thumb, tape it with 3–4 figure-eight patterns around the joint. **OR** —keeping hand and fingers in the position of function (cupping shape as though holding a baseball) with extra padding in the palm. Secure the hand, fingers, and arm to a splint. (See Appendix B for instructions on how to apply a Sam® Splint to a finger.) 5. Place arm in a sling and swathe (binder).

Finger Injury Care (continued)

IF . . .	THEN . . .
	6. Treat for shock by keeping the athlete warm and lying down with straight legs elevated 8–12 inches.
	7. Seek immediate medical attention.
	Improper care of a dislocation, especially the thumb, can cause more damage (to nerves and blood vessels) than that of the initial injury.

UPPER

Finger Injury Care (continued)

IF . . .	THEN . . .

finger or thumb has been:
• "jammed" or compressed
• stepped on
• forced or twisted sideways
AND athlete has:
• pain and is unable to make a fist
• pain which radiates from injury site when gentle pressure is applied to area—or if finger tip is pushed/pulled to/from wrist
• weakness while curling injured finger alone
• weakness or pain with grip
	suspect a significant *contusion, sprain,* or *possible fracture:*
	1. Apply an ice pack for 20–30 minutes.
	2. Reevaluate after completion of ice pack application:
	   —Seek medical evaluation prior to athlete's returning to participation if pain and weakness exist.
	   —Return to participation is possible if area is painless to touch and motion is painless.
	3. Tape fingers with "buddy" taping for support. Tape thumb with 3–4 figure-eight patterns around joint.
	4. Apply an ice pack 3–4 times, for 20–30 minutes each time, through first 48 hours.

U
P
P
E
R

Finger Injury Care (continued)

IF . . .	THEN . . .
	5. Seek medical evaluation if pain or swelling increases within first 24 hours.
fingernail was hit or stepped on and blood is seen under the nail **AND** • is painful because of blood build-up under nail	suspect a *blood clot* exists under nail: 1. Apply an ice pack while elevating the hand or place finger in ice water for 10 minutes. 2. Depending upon situation, it may be necessary to seek medical attention.
fingernail is partially torn loose	take the following precautions: 1. Do *not* remove the nail. 2. Return nail to normal position. 3. Apply antibiotic ointment, dressing, and bandage. 4. For large area, seek medical attention.

U
P
P
E
R

Finger Injury Care (continued)

IF . . .	THEN . . .
fingernail is completely torn off	proceed as follows: 1. Apply antibiotic ointment over area. 2. Apply dressing and bandage. 3. Seek medical attention.

U
P
P
E
R

Injuries to the
Lower Extremities

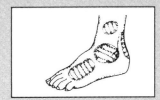

Thigh Injuries

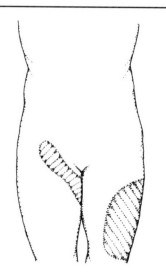

The thigh consists of a single bone, the femur, which is surrounded and protected by heavy muscle. The muscle group on the front of the thigh is the "quadriceps group." Most thigh injuries are from direct trauma or excessive torsion. Much like other leg muscles, a quadriceps strain can happen early in the season or if the athlete is not adequately warmed up for participation.

Thigh Injury Care

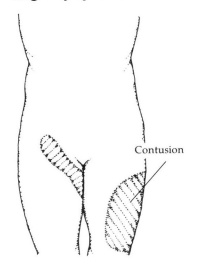

Contusion

If athlete . . .	THEN . . .
received a direct hit producing: • swelling • pain and tenderness • firmness of site when pressed • visible bruise which may appear hours later	suspect a *muscle contusion* (*bruising*): 1. Follow RICE procedures as explained in Appendix A. 2. Stretch muscle by bending knee toward athlete's chest. 3. Apply an ice pack for 20–30 minutes, 3–4 times daily for next 48 hours. 4. Do ***not*** apply heat.

L
O
W
E
R

Thigh Injury Care (continued)

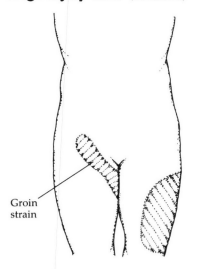

Groin strain

If athlete . . .	THEN . . .
while running or jumping: • feels popping or pulling **AND** later has: • tenderness • stiffness and pain during leg movement • swelling • visible bruise which may appear days later	suspect a *muscle strain* (*tear*): 1. Follow RICE procedures as explained in Appendix A. 2. Keep injured muscle stretched. 3. Apply an ice pack for 20–30 minutes, 3–4 times daily for next 48 hours. 4. Do *not* apply heat.

LOWER

Hamstring Injuries

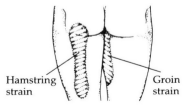

Hamstring strain

Groin strain

A hamstring injury can be a strain including a tear in the muscle. This type of injury is due to explosive movement, such as sprinting or acceleration while running. As with other leg muscle injuries, a hamstring strain can result if the athlete is not adequately warmed up, or can occur early in the season.

Hamstring Injury Care

IF . . .	THEN . . .
while running or jumping, athlete: • feels a pop or pulling sensation at back of thigh **AND** at the time of injury has: • tenderness to touch • swelling • stiffness or pain when bending knee or trying to touch toes	suspect *muscle strain* (*tear*): 1. Use RICE procedures explained in Appendix A. 2. Wrap compression pad under elastic bandage. 3. Wake athlete during the first night after the injury to gently stretch. 4. Keep muscle stretched; do *not* force stretching.

Hamstring Injury Care (continued)

IF . . .	THEN . . .
athlete has no pain bending knee and touching toes while sitting **AND** can run painlessly without a limp: • forward/backward • cutting and changing direction • in figure eights • in any other direction necessary for functional participation	in order for athlete to return to participation 1. Support area with wrap or sleeve. 2. Maintain ice pack application for 20–30 minutes, 3–4 times daily during first 48 hours. 3. Maintain full flexibility without forcing stretching.

Knee Injuries

Knee injuries are amongst the most serious joint injuries in athletic participation, and can cause the athlete a high level of anxiety. Their severity is difficult to determine, thus a thorough medical evaluation is necessary if the injury is traumatic and not from overuse. Athletes in running and jumping sports may devlop some chronic soreness, particularly early in the season.

Knee Injury Care

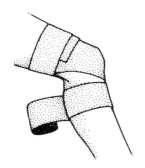

IF . . .	THEN . . .
at the time of injury, the athlete has • pain • feeling of a pop or snap • locking sensation • unusual, obvious deformity **OR** athlete • may not be able to walk without limping • may not be able to bend or straighten knee	suspect *sprain with internal damage,* or *possible fracture:* 1. Remove clothing from knee. If knee is obviously dislocated, do **not** force into place. Splint knee in position found and seek immediate medical attention. (See Appendix B for instructions on how to apply a Sam® Splint to an injured knee.) 2. Apply RICE procedures explained in Appendix A. 3. Seek medical evaluation prior to a return to participation.

Knee Injury Care (continued)

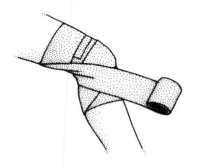

IF . . .	THEN . . .
after comparison to healthy knee, athlete has: • pain when straightening or bending injured knee • tenderness or pain when pressing the area of damage • inability to bear weight on the injured leg alone • apprehension about crouching into a baseball catcher's squat	suspect a *sprain with questionable damage:* 1. Follow RICE procedures explained in Appendix A; crutches recommended. 2. Seek medical attention prior to allowing athlete to return to participation. 3. Monitor swelling; significant ligament injuries have more swelling 24 hours after the injury than at the time of injury.

LOWER

Knee Injury Care (continued)

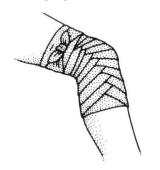

IF . . .	THEN . . .
athlete is able to bear weight on single leg and can run at normal speed and without a limp: • forward/backward • in figure eights • cutting and changing direction	suspect *mild sprain:* 1. Follow RICE procedures explained in Appendix A. 2. Athlete's return to participation is possible with adequate taping or bracing, but a medical evaluation is recommended.
pain is chronic or ongoing, caused by running or jumping **AND:** • increases during activity • kneecap is sore to probing or gentle pressure • muscles around kneecap feel weak	suspect *overuse injury:* 1. Apply heat before activity. 2. Apply an ice pack after activity. 3. Seek medical attention for appropriate rehabilitation program and supportive sleeve or brace.

Knee Injury Care (continued)

IF . . .	THEN . . .
after a direct blow to the kneecap athlete has: • pain • swelling • tenderness • bruise marks (black-and-blue discoloration)	suspect a *contusion* (*bruised knee*): 1. Follow RICE procedures explained in Appendix A.
After a single blow or repeated impacts athlete has: • moderate pain • a kneecap that feels squishy	suspect *traumatic bursitis* (*water on the knee*): 1. Follow RICE procedures explained in Appendix A. 2. Fluid can be drained by physician in case of severe injury.

LOWER

Knee Injury Care (continued)

IF . . .	THEN . . .
knee was twisted or wrenched and athlete • felt it "give way," snap, and "lock" or not move • experiences pain • is unable to completely bend or straighten knee	suspect *cartilage (meniscus) injury:* 1. Follow RICE procedures explained in Appendix A. 2. Seek medical attention.
after a blow to the knee or twisting of knee athlete feels: • "pop" • pain • swelling • loose sensation	suspect *ligament injury:* 1. Follow RICE procedures explained in Appendix A. 2. Seek medical attention.

Knee Injury Care (continued)

IF . . .	THEN . . .
a blow or twisting causes kneecap to be moved to the outside of the knee joint and there is: • possible swelling • inability to bend or straighten knee • pain • deformity	suspect *dislocated kneecap:* 1. Follow RICE procedures explained in Appendix A. 2. Do not try to relocate a dislocated kneecap (sometimes the kneecap replaces itself). 3. Seek medical attention.
after a major blow to the leg or a sudden, forceful twist, the knee has: • excruciating pain • deformity • no pulse is felt in the leg (feel for pulse at the groove between the Achilles tendon and the inside ankle-knob bone, i.e., the tibia)	suspect a *dislocated knee joint:* 1. Immediately seek medical attention.
Do NOT move an injured knee in an attempt to determine the type of knee injury or whether the injury is minor or severe. More damage can happen. Such testing requires years of training.	

L
O
W
E
R

Shin (Front of Lower Leg) Injuries

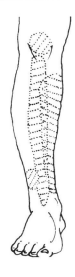

The two bones of the lower leg are the tibia (larger) and fibula (smaller). Most shin injuries are "shin splints," which are strains from overuse, such as running or jumping. Occasionally, a bone is fractured from overuse.

Shin Injury Care

IF . . .	THEN . . .
athlete receives hit directly on shin and has: • tenderness to touch • sharp pain **BUT** later has: • an abnormal tingling running up and down shin • difficulty moving ankle up and down • numbness or coldness in toes or foot	suspect *contusion:* 1. Apply RICE procedures explained in Appendix A, utilizing a compression wrap. Use an ice pack for 20–30 minutes, 3–4 times daily for first 48 hours. 2. Athlete's return to participation is based on level of pain and ability to bear weight on leg and function adequately. 3. If numbness or tingling is noted, prompt medical attention is necessary.

Shin Injury Care (continued)

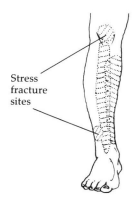

Stress
fracture
sites

IF . . .	THEN . . .
pain over bone is chronic and: • is evident during activity • does not subside after activity is stopped • is evident while sleeping • is localized to the size of 50-cent piece	suspect *stress fracture:* 1. Apply RICE procedures explained in Appendix A. 2. Seek medical attention. 3. Athlete's return to participation is based on medical evaluation.

Shin Injury Care (continued)

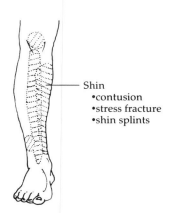

Shin
- contusion
- stress fracture
- shin splints

IF . . .	THEN . . .
shin aches during activity, but: • ache subsides significantly after activity stops • ache is result of increase in workout routine (e.g., running longer, running on hills, etc.)	suspect "*shin splints*": 1. Apply an ice pack before activity. Heat can be applied later, when the athlete is well on the way to recovery. 2. Use one of several taping methods: —Use X-arch taping to support arches (1-inch or 1½-inch athlete tape and underwrap). —Apply pressure with a 3-inch elastic wrap over sorest point (start below sore area and spiral wrap up and around leg). 3. Apply an ice pack for 30 minutes after activity. 4. Curtail activity until pain-free.

L
O
W
E
R

Shin Injury Care (continued)

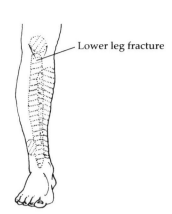

Lower leg fracture

IF . . .	THEN . . .
a direct blow or twisting forces produce: • severe pain • swelling • visible deformity • tenderness to the touch	suspect a *lower leg fracture:* 1. Follow RICE procedures explained in Appendix A. 2. Stabilize injured leg using an improvised splint or a Sam® Splint (see Appendix B). 3. Seek medical attention.

Calf and Achilles Tendon Injuries

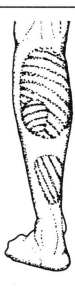

The Achilles tendon is the thick band in the back of the leg that connects the two calf muscles (gastrocnemius and soleus) to the heel. Injuries to the muscle can be from a direct trauma or torsion strain. A strain is generally found in sports involving jumping, running, explosive starts and stops, and direction changes. A rupture, or complete tear, of the Achilles tendon is uncommon, but can occur during one of these explosive activities.

Calf and Achilles Tendon Injury Care

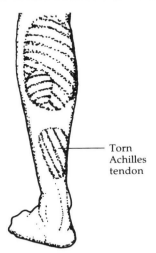

Torn Achilles tendon

If athlete . . .	THEN . . .
feels a "pop" within the Achilles tendon which produces: • constant pain or pain with movement • tenderness to touch • inability to bear weight on injured leg • "crackling" feeling and sound **OR** if athlete: • can't push up on toes • has difficulty in controlling foot (foot flops around)	suspect a *torn Achilles tendon:* 1. Apply RICE procedures explained in Appendix A. 2. Place athlete on crutches and seek medical attention. 3. Pad heels of both feet to reduce stress. 4. Seek medical attention prior to returning to participation.

L
O
W
E
R

Calf and Achilles Tendon Injury Care (continued)

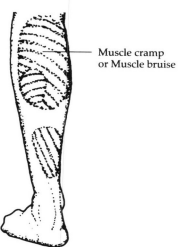

Muscle cramp
or Muscle bruise

IF . . .	THEN . . .
receives direct hit producing: • swelling • pain and tenderness while moving ankle up and down • feeling of firmness when area is pressed	suspect *muscle contusion (bruise)*: 1. Apply an ice pack 20–30 minutes, 3–4 times daily during first 48 hours. 2. Use compression with elastic bandage holding pressure pad. 3. Maintain as much pain-free flexibility as possible. Do *not* force stretching.

Calf and Achilles Tendon Injury Care (continued)

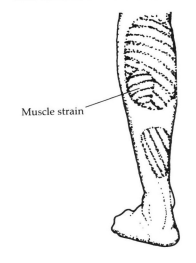

Muscle strain

IF . . .	THEN . . .
while running or jumping: • feels pop or pulling in muscle in back of leg and behind knee **AND** later has: • tenderness • stiffness and pain while moving ankle up and down • swelling	suspect *muscle strain (tear):* 1. Follow instructions regarding the application of an ice pack and compression explained above. 2. Do *not* return to activity until tenderness/stiffness diminishes and allows movement.
experiences: • pain occurring just above the heel • pain while jumping and/or running	suspect *Achilles tendinitis:* 1. Apply an ice pack for 15–20 minutes, 3–4 times daily. 2. Rest from activity. 3. Elevate heel with heel cup, pads, or wedges in shoes.

Calf and Achilles Tendon Injury Care (continued)

IF . . .	THEN . . .
is able to: • bear weight on injured foot and raise onto toes • run forward and backward at normal speed without pain or a limp • run with change of direction at normal speed without pain or a limp • demonstrate normal flexibility	allow a return to participation: 1. Apply heat before activity. 2. Wrap, brace, or tape the area for support. 3. Apply ice pack after activity. 4. Seek medical attention for appropriate rehabilitation program.

LOWER

Calf and Achilles Tendon Injury Care (continued)

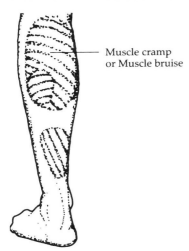

Muscle cramp or Muscle bruise

IF . . .	THEN . . .
calf muscle has: • extremely painful cramp or spasm • disables athlete	suspect a *muscle cramp:* 1. Gently stretch the calf muscle by having the athlete sit with the leg straight. The coach should gently press the foot toward the shin for about 1 minute and then slowly release **OR** 2. Gently stretch the muscle by having the athlete stand with both feet on the floor, with the affected leg in the rear. Bend the front leg to stretch the rear leg's calf muscle, keeping the rear foot flat on the floor and the rear leg straight. **OR**

L
O
W
E
R

Calf and Achilles Tendon Injury Care (continued)

IF . . .	THEN . . .
	3. Apply hand pressure to the affected muscle (do not massage). **OR**
	4. Apply an ice pack to the cramped muscle because it causes the muscles to relax. The exception to this might be during cold weather.
	5. Pinch the upper lip hard (an acupressure technique).
	6. Do *not* give salt tablets (they can draw fluid out of the circulatory system and into the stomach).
	7. Drink water, since fluid deficiency appears to be the main cause of a muscle cramp. Avoid drinks with too much sugar since they don't leave the stomach quickly.

L
O
W
E
R

Calf and Achilles Tendon Injury Care (continued)

IF . . .	THEN . . .
	8. Allow athlete to return to participation based on: —the ability to bear weight painlessly on leg—both flat-footed and on toes —the ability to run: • forward/backward • in figure eights • in changing directions.

Ankle Injury

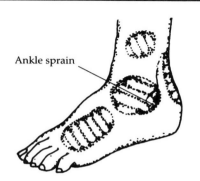

Ankle sprain

Most ankle injuries are sprains; about 85% of sprains involve the ankle's outside (lateral) ligaments and are caused by having the ankle turned/twisted inward. If improperly treated, a sprained ankle becomes chronically susceptible for future sprains.

Ankle Injury Care

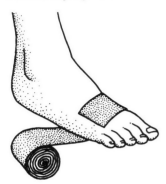

If the injured athlete has . . .	THEN . . .
at the time of injury: • pain • feeling of popping or tearing **AND** later, when compared with the healthy ankle, the injured ankle has: • loss of use • swelling • tenderness or pain when you press above, below, and to the sides of the injury site	suspect a *sprain:* 1. Take off the athlete's shoe and sock. 2. Do *not* move or test the laxity of the ankle. All ankle sprains and fractures can receive the same initial treatment.

Ankle Injury Care

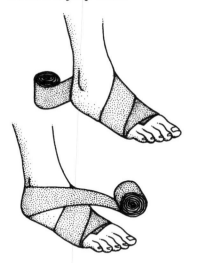

If the injured athlete has . . .	THEN . . .
	3. Follow RICE procedures (see also Appendix A): —**R**est means no weight on the ankle. —**I**ce (crushed) should be applied for 20–30 minutes every 2–3 hours during the next 48 hours. Crushed ice fits the body's contours better. Protect the skin with a single layer of loosely applied elastic wrap placed between the ice bag and the skin. The rest of the elastic wrap can be used to hold the ice bag in place.

LOWER

Ankle Injury Care (continued)

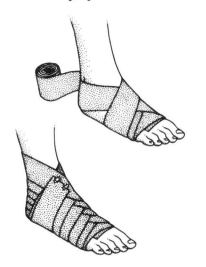

If the injured athlete has . . .	THEN . . .
	—Compression is achieved by applying an elastic bandage over a ½-inch thick felt horseshoe padding or by using any soft pliable material (e.g., the athlete's own sock or T-shirt) placed in a "U" shape around the ankle knob with the curved part down.
	—Elevation means keeping the injured ankle at or above waist level at all times when not using it. Continue both compression and elevation until swelling is gone.

Ankle Injury Care (continued)

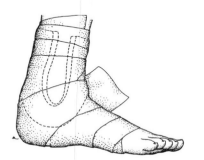

If the injured athlete has . . .	THEN . . .
	4. Seek medical evaluation prior to return to participation.

Ankle Injury Care (continued)

If the injured athlete has . . .	THEN . . .
• an unusual deformity in the injured ankle compared with the healthy ankle • refused to put any weight on the injured foot • placed weight on the injured foot and feels something grinding or gravelly • hopped off the field or court on the good leg, but complains that it hurts the injured ankle • a numb feeling or tingling, or foot feels cold • pain/tenderness radiating to or from the injury when you press around the injury site • swelling, which may appear on both sides of the ankle	—suspect a *fracture:* 1. For ankle injuries, use the **RICE** procedure described above and in Appendix A. 2. Stabilize ankle with pillow or folded blanket. 3. Seek medical attention.

Ankle Injury Care (continued)

- The amount of swelling and pain does not indicate the injury's severity.
- **Avoid** applying heat to the injured ankle for at least 48 hours after the injury.
- Seek medical attention for ankle fractures, dislocations, severe sprains, and sprains affecting the ankle's ligaments.

LOWER

Foot Injury

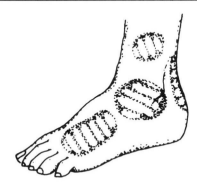

Foot injuries are common in sports because of the foot's role in bearing weight. Foot sprains, strains, and fractures can be traumatic in nature, or chronic, such as arch strain. Some foot injuries may not disable an athlete, but will limit their best efforts.

Foot Injury Care

IF . . .	THEN . . .
at the time of injury, the foot has: • severe pain **AND** later, when compared to healthy foot, it has: • swelling • visible deformity • tenderness around injury site when gently probed • pain radiating from injury site when gently probed • numbness and cold feeling • loss of use (i.e., inability to use or pain when bearing weight)	suspect possible *fracture* or *sprain:* 1. Follow RICE procedures explained in Appendix A. 2. Treat for shock, if needed. 3. If pain persists, seek medical evaluation before athlete's return to participation. 4. Place athlete on crutches, if needed.

LOWER

Foot Injury Care (continued)

IF . . .	THEN . . .
toe(s) have: • severe pain • swelling • visible deformity in some cases • pain and tenderness to touch • pain or inability to use when bearing weight • loss of use or range of motion	suspect possible *fracture* or *sprain:* 1. Follow RICE procedures explained in Appendix A. 2. Using "buddy" method, tape toe to adjacent uninjured toe with something absorbent between the toes to absorb perspiration. 3. Seek medical evaluation before athlete's return to participation. 4. Use crutches, if needed.

Foot Injury Care (continued)

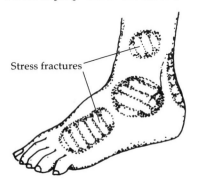

Stress fractures

IF . . .	THEN . . .
pain occcurs, is chronic, and: • is evident during activity • does not stop after completion of activity • is localized (affected area is about the size of a dime or nickel) at the site of a bump over a bone • swelling occurs over painful site	suspect possible *stress fracture:* 1. Apply an ice pack to injury for 20–30 minutes. 2. Stop all activity. 3. Apply "doughnut pad" over area to relieve pressure. 4. Seek medical evaluation before athlete's return to participation.

LOWER

Foot Injury Care (continued)

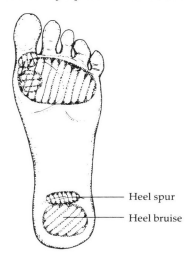

Heel spur
Heel bruise

IF . . .	THEN . . .
pain occurs at bottom of heel and: • soreness relates to change in participation routine (i.e., increased running time or distance; running uphill and downhill; hard surface jumping, etc.) • pain has been gradual in nature	suspect *heel bruise, heel spur,* or *strained arch:* 1. Apply an ice pack after activity for 20–30 minutes, 3–4 times daily. 2. Support area with rigid plastic heel cup or taping procedure. 3. Seek medical evaluation to establish exact diagnosis and treatment.

Foot Injury Care (continued)

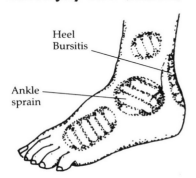

Heel
Bursitis

Ankle
sprain

IF . . .	THEN . . .
pain occurs at back of heel in area where shoe rubs (resembles Achilles tendinitis)	suspect *inflammation* (*bursitis*): 1. Apply an ice pack for 15–20 minutes, or ice massage for 5–7 minutes, 3–4 times daily. 2. Apply a "doughnut pad" or other padding over area to distribute pain which is producing the friction. 3. Bend the back of the athlete's shoe several times to make it more flexible. 4. Rest if inflammation disrupts normal participation and seek medical evaluation for appropriate treatment.

Foot Injury Care (continued)

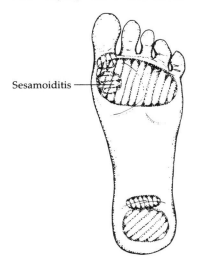

Sesamoiditis

IF . . .	THEN . . .
pain occurs under the ball of the foot at the big toe and if this spot hurts when you press on the ball of the foot and pull back on the big toe to stretch the tendon	suspect *sesamoiditis:* 1. Apply an ice pack for 20–30 minutes, 3–4 times daily. 2. Put a small pad below the area to reduce the pounding on the affected area. 3. If pain persists, seek medical evaluation.

Foot Injury Care (continued)

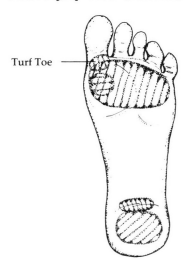

Turf Toe

IF . . .	THEN . . .
pain and swelling occur at the base of the big toe (may involve other toes) when stepping forward or landing on toes	suspect *turf toe:* 1. Apply an ice pack for 15–20 minutes, 3–4 times daily. 2. "Buddy" tape affected toe(s) to one uninjured. 3. Place stiff insert into shoe to decrease its flexibility. 4. If pain persists, seek medical attention.

L
O
W
E
R

Foot Injury Care (continued)

IF . . .	THEN . . .
no evidence of fracture exists and athlete can do the following without pain: • bear weight on injured foot alone • stand on toes with weight evenly distributed on both feet • complete 5 "jumping jacks" with feet landing together • run forward/backward • hop on injured foot • run figure eights at normal speed without a limp • perform any activity specific to the type of sports participation	consider athlete's resuming participation: 1. Apply an ice pack after activity if soreness exists. 2. Support injured area with appropriate taping, bracing, or padding as needed. 3. Seek medical evaluation if chronic pain returns soon after activity has resumed.

Blisters

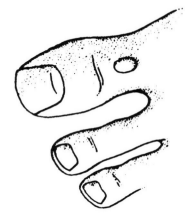

Blister Care

IF . . .	THEN . . .
area on skin is a "hot spot" (painful, red area)	1. Cool "hot spot" with an ice pack or soaking in ice water. 2. Apply lubrication ointment or petroleum jelly over irritated area. **OR** 3. Tape a gauze pad or bandage strip over ointment or petroleum jelly—or use a felt (moleskin) doughnut pad as described below. **OR** 4. Cover it with Spenco Second Skin™ (a slippery pad) which will absorb the friction.
blister is torn and fluid or blood is seeping or flowing out	1. Clean it with disinfectant. 2. Follow treatment procedures for open blister described below.

- 185 -

Blister Care (continued)

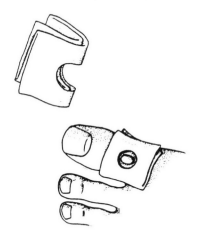

IF . . .	THEN . . .
blister on foot is closed	1. Cut a hole in a piece of moleskin to fit around blister.
	2. Apply thin layer of lubricant over blister, or use Spenco Second Skin™.
	3. Place moleskin with hole over blister.
	4. Put gauze pad over lubricant and moleskin.
	5. Tape moleskin-gauze pad unit to foot.
	6. Continue the above care until blister is healed.

LOWER

Blister Care (continued)

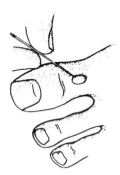

IF . . .	THEN . . .
blister on foot is open, or a very painful closed blister affects walking/running	1. Drain all fluid out of blister while wearing gloves. 2. Trim blister's roof edge with sterilized biological scissors. Use tweezers to lift up blister's roof. 3. Clean affected area with disinfectant. 4. Apply antibiotic (e.g., Polysporin™ or Neosporin™) ointment. 5. Duplicate procedures listed above for treating a closed blister and apply a pad to protect blister. 6. Continue the above care until blister is healed. 7. Watch for signs of infection (pus, increased pain, redness). Seek medical attention if infection develops.

Calluses/Corns/ Athlete's Foot

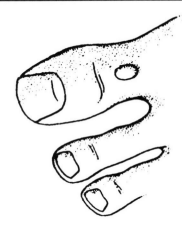

Skin problems are common in athletes because of the skin's large surface area, perspiration, friction, and the many pathogens in the athletic environment.

Calluses/Corns/Athlete's Foot Care

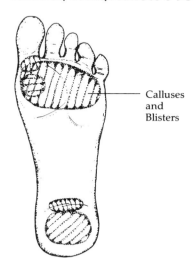

Calluses and Blisters

If a painless mass of dead skin appears from chronic irritation . . .	THEN . . .
	suspect a *callus:* 1. Soak area in warm water to make skin pliable. 2. Dry skin thoroughly. Use a standard emery board, sandpaper, or a commercial callus file to rub callus down until it is as smooth as skin surrounding it. Do *not* cut with a razor. 3. Soften skin with lubricant.

Calluses/Corns/Athlete's Foot Care (continued)

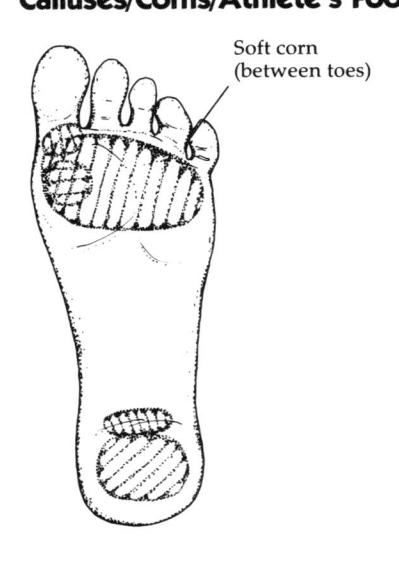

Soft corn (between toes)

If a painful callus . . .	THEN . . .
appears on top of toes	suspect a *"hard"* corn: 1. Take pressure off site using a felt doughnut or horseshoe pad with tape over it. 2. Only a physician should remove a corn.
appears between toes	suspect a *"soft"* corn: 1. Wash in soap and water and dry thoroughly. 2. Insert small piece of lamb's wool between toes to allow drying. 3. Do *not* use commercial corn-removal preparations.

L
O
W
E
R

Calluses/Corns/Athlete's Foot Care (continued)

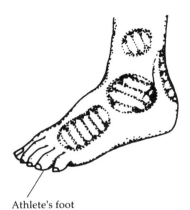

Athlete's foot

IF . . .	THEN . . .
a red, scaly rash appears around toes that is accompanied by burning and itching	suspect *athlete's foot:* 1. Have athlete keep feet dry by changing socks daily. 2. Have athlete use foot powder to absorb sweat. 3. Have athlete apply antifungal cream to area (e.g., Tinactin,™ Micatin™). 4. Seek medical attention if the above procedures fail to work.

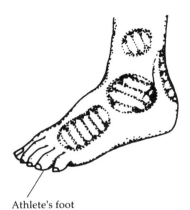

Environment-related Emergencies

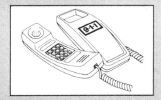

Sunburn

It is difficult to accurately gauge the amount of ultraviolet light the skin has received. It is not until hours after exposure that the sunburned skin confirms the athlete's error of staying too long exposed to the sun. Sunburn can be a first- or second-degree burn.

Sunburn Care

IF . . .	THEN . . .
• redness appears immediately after exposure and starts to disappear after 30 minutes, and 2–6 hours later delayed redness can be seen, peaking at 10–24 hours, with fading over the next 2–4 days, a first-degree sunburn is indicated • blisters and pain occur, this usually indicates a second-degree sunburn	take the following precautions: 1. Avoid any further exposure to the sun. 2. If eyes have been affected, seek medical attention. 3. Cool affected area with cold tap water (which is usually 70–75°F). Tissue retains heat and may continue burning for up to 20 minutes after exposure. Cool water eliminates heat, limits damage, and gives pain relief. Apply cold for up to 30 minutes.

E
N
V
I
R
O
N

Sunburn Care (continued)

IF . . .	THEN . . .
Complications of severe sunburn include: • dehydration (excessive loss of water from the body) • fever, chills, and nausea • intense pain • heat-related injuries (heat stroke and heat exhaustion) • broken blisters	4. Do *not* apply ice directly to the skin because frostbite may result. However, for some body locations (i.e., face) or when there is no water, an ice pack wrapped in a damp cloth can provide relief. Do *not* apply ice directly to the skin or for over 20–30 minutes. 5. If blisters appear within 2–3 days, do not break them. If they break, wash the area with water, pat dry, and cover with dry, sterile gauze to prevent infection. Peeling can happen anywhere from 4–7 days.

Sunburn Care (continued)

IF . . .	THEN . . .
	6. Do *not* use over-the-counter topical burn ointments or sprays because: —Some may cause an allergic reaction. —Most do not contain enough benzocaine or lidocaine to depress pain. —Duration of any possible relief is relatively short (30–40 minutes). More than 3 or 4 applications per day of products containing local anesthetics is discouraged because toxicity can occur if these agents are used too frequently. —They seal in the heat. 7. Do *not* use butter, lard, or petroleum jelly.

Sunburn Care (continued)

IF . . .	THEN . . .
	8. For burned legs and swollen feet, elevate the legs above the heart level.
	9. Have athlete drink lots of water to counteract the drying effect of a burn.
	10. For first-degree burns, keep the skin moistened.
	11. Do *not* use aloe vera until after applying cold to the area and the pain has stopped. Test a small area of sunburned skin first to make sure the athlete is not allergic to aloe vera.

ENVIRON

Sunburn Care (continued)

IF . . .	THEN . . .
	12. Soothe sunburn after the initial cold treatment with: —Aveeno Bath Treatment (½ cup), which is made from oatmeal, added to a tub of cool water; soak the athlete for 15–20 minutes. —Baking soda (½ cup) sprinkled into bathwater; allow it to dry on the skin. 13. Excessive sun exposure may be associated with heat exhaustion and heat stroke. Refer to the following section on heat-related emergencies for more information.

E
N
V
I
R
O
N

Heat-related Emergencies

Athletes are especially susceptible to heat-related illnesses. These illness are most common in football, but can occur in any sport and are easily prevented. Coaches and athletic trainers should enforce adequate water intake. These illnesses happen most often when athletes exercise in a hot, humid environment. It is important to remember that a "heat stroke" is a medical emergency and requires emergency medical attention. Refer to the "heat index" table.

Heat Related Emergency Care

If athlete, while exposed to warm/hot environment, has . . .	THEN . . .
• rectal body temperature over 105°F (oral and armpit readings are not as accurate as rectal reading) • rapid breathing and pulse • completely disoriented • become unresponsive • experienced a seizure • sweaty, wet skin • ashen, gray skin color	suspect *heat stroke:* • *Exertional heat stroke* affects the healthy athlete when he/she is playing strenuously or working in a warm environment. **Immediately call the EMS system and:** 1. Monitor the ABCs (airway, breathing, and circulation) and treat accordingly. 2. Move athlete to cool place and remove excess clothing.

E
N
V
I
R
O
N

Heat Related Emergency Care (continued)

If athlete, while exposed to warm/hot environment, has ...	THEN ...
	3. Immediately cool athlete by wrapping him/her in wet towels or sheets and fanning athlete; or place ice packs on areas with abundant blood supply (e.g., neck, armpits, groin).
	4. Monitor rectal temperature every 5–10 minutes and stop cooling when body temperature reaches 103°F.
	5. Keep head and shoulders slightly elevated.
	6. Care for seizures if they occur.

Heat Related Emergency Care (continued)

If athlete while exposed to warm/hot environment has . . .	THEN . . .
• heavy sweating • weakness • fast pulse • normal body temperature • headache and dizziness • nausea and vomiting	suspect *heat exhaustion:* 1. Move athlete to a cool place. 2. Have athlete lie down with straight legs elevated. 3. Cool by applying cold pack or wet towels or cloths over athlete, as well as by fanning. 4. Give athlete cold water to drink if he/she is conscious. 5. Seek medical attention before allowing athlete to return to participation.

E
N
V
I
R
O
N

Heat Related Emergency Care (continued)

If athlete while exposed to warm/hot environment has . . .	THEN . . .
• severe cramping or muscle spasms which affect legs or arms • abdominal cramping	suspect a *heat cramp:* 1. Move athlete to a cool place. 2. Have athlete rest the cramping muscle. 3. Have athlete drink a lot of cold water. 4. Do *not* massage affected muscle. 5. Try the acupressure method of pinching the upper lip for relief.

Table 10-1 / Effect of relative humidity on air temperature

					Air Temperature						
	70	75	80	85	90	95	100	105	110	115	120
Relative Humidity					Apparent Temperature*						
0%	64	69	73	78	83	87	91	95	99	103	107
10%	65	70	75	80	85	90	95	100	105	111	116
20%	66	72	77	82	87	93	99	105	112	120	130
30%	67	73	78	84	90	96	104	113	123	135	148
40%	68	74	79	86	93	101	110	123	137	151	
50%	69	75	81	88	96	107	120	135	150		
60%	70	76	82	90	100	114	132	149			
70%	70	77	85	93	106	124	144				
80%	71	78	86	97	113	136					
90%	71	79	88	102	122						
100%	72	80	91	108							

*Degrees Fahrenheit.

Above 130°F = heat stroke imminent
105°–130°F = heat exhaustion and heat cramps likely; heat stroke with long exposure and activity
90°–105°F = heat exhaustion and heat cramps with long exposure and activity
80°–90°F = fatigue during exposure and activity

Source: National Weather Service

Frostbite

Frostbite happens when outside air temperatures drop below freezing (32°F) and the skin's tissue freezes. It mainly affects the feet, hands, ears, and nose. Depending on the temperature and wind velocity, frostbite can happen in a short period of time. Refer to the "wind chill factor" table.

Frostbite Care

If an athlete has been exposed to freezing temperatures (below 32°F) and has . . .	THEN . . .
• skin color becoming lighter (blanching or turning white or pale) • a body part which feels numb but is not painful	suspect *frostnip*, which is not serious, but warns that frostbite can happen with continued exposure to freezing temperatures: 1. Treat by gently rewarming affected area by either: 　—using bare hands on area 　—blowing warm air on area 　—if hands are affected, placing them in armpits. 2. During rewarming, stinging, tingling, or burning sensations may occur. 3. Suspect frostbite if area does *not* respond.

E
N
V
I
R
O
N

Frostbite Care (continued)

If an athlete has been exposed to freezing temperatures (below 32°F) and has . . .	THEN . . .
• skin color which appears white, waxy, or grayish-yellow • pain which is felt initially, but later quits • said area feels cold and numb (may also complain of tingling and stinging sensations) • skin surface which feels hard or crusty and underlying tissue is soft when depressed gently and firmly	suspect *superficial frostbite,* which is serious. Severity of frostbite varies from superficial to deep. Regardless of severity, treat all frostbite the same: 1. Rewarming seldom takes place outside of a medical facility because such facilities are usually nearby. 2. When medical care is delayed, put affected body part in warm (not hot) water. Test the water by sprinkling some on the inside of your arm.

E
N
V
I
R
O
N

Frostbite Care (continued)

If an athlete has been exposed to freezing temperatures (below 32°F) and has . . .	THEN . . .
Note: Deep frostbite is *not* discussed since athletes are not likely victims. All frostbite—superficial or deep—is treated the same.	3. Rewarming usually takes 20–40 minutes and should be continued until tissues are soft and pliable. 4. For ear or facial areas, apply warm, moist cloths and change them frequently to keep them warm. 5. Dry rewarming (e.g., hands in armpits) takes 3–4 times longer than the wet method, resulting in greater tissue damage. 6. Do *not* allow body part to freeze again after thawing since greater damage results (because larger ice crystals will be formed).

E
N
V
I
R
O
N

Frostbite Care (continued)

If an athlete has been exposed to freezing temperatures (below 32°F) and has . . .	THEN . . .
	7. Do *not* break any blisters that may be formed.
	8. Do *not* rub the body part. Do *not* rub the body part with snow.
	9. Do *not* allow athlete to walk on frostbitten toes or feet, especially after rewarming.
	10. Elevate injured body part to reduce pain and swelling.
	11. After thawing, place dry, sterile gauze between toes and fingers to absorb moisture and avoid having them stick together.
	12. Keep athlete warm.
	13. Seek immediate medical attention.

E
N
V
I
R
O
N

Hypothermia	Hypothermia (low temperature) happens when the body temperature falls below 95°F. The athlete's body cannot produce enough energy to keep the internal (core) temperature at a satisfactory level.

Hypothermia happens mainly in winter, but can also happen in temperatures as high as 50°F. Athletes become susceptible to hypothermia when they have inadequate or wet clothing.

Hypothermia

If athlete is exposed to cold temperatures (they do not have to be below freezing) and has . . .	THEN . . .
• shivering • slurred speech • memory lapses • fumbling hands • stumbling and staggering • cold hands, feet, abdomen, and back	suspect *mild hypothermia:* In order to stop further heat loss: 1. Move athlete to warm place. 2. Add insulation around athlete. Cover athlete's head, since 50% of the body's heat is lost through the head. 3. Replace wet clothing (may be damp from perspiration and/or wet weather) with dry clothing. 4. Place warm packs against the body's areas of high heat loss (e.g., head, neck, chest, and groin). Do *not* burn athlete. 5. Seek immediate medical attention.

Hypothermia (continued)

If athlete is exposed to cold temperatures (they do not have to be below freezing) and has . . .	THEN . . .
	Caution: 1. Handle athlete very gently, as though every arm and leg were broken. 2. Do *not* rub arms and legs. 3. Do *not* rewarm extremities and body core (chest, abdomen) at the same time.

E
N
V
I
R
O
N

Hypothermia (continued)

If athlete has . . .	THEN . . .
• had previous shivering that has stopped • stiff and rigid muscles (similar to rigor mortis) • skin with blue appearance • slow pulse and breathing • dilated pupils • become unconscious (appears dead)	suspect *profound hypothermia. This condition will rarely be seen in athletes. In order to treat:* 1. Move athlete out of the cold. 2. Handle athlete very gently, as though every arm and leg were broken. 3. Do *not* rewarm athlete (this should take place only in a medical facility). 4. Do *not* rub legs or arms. 5. Seek immediate medical attention.

E
N
V
I
R
O
N

Table 10-2 / Wind-Chill Factor

Estimated Wind Speed (in MPH)	Actual Thermometer Reading (°F)											
	50	40	30	20	10	0	−10	−20	−30	−40	−50	−60
	Equivalent Temperature (°F)											
calm	50	40	30	20	10	0	−10	−20	−30	−40	−50	−60
5	48	37	27	16	6	−5	−15	−26	−36	−47	−57	−68
10	40	28	16	4	−9	−24	−33	−46	−58	−70	−83	−95
15	36	22	9	−5	−18	−32	−45	−58	−72	−85	−99	−112
20	32	18	4	−10	−25	−39	−53	−67	−82	−96	−110	−124
25	30	16	0	−15	−29	−44	−59	−74	−88	−104	−118	−133
30	25	13	−2	−18	−33	−48	−63	−79	−94	−109	−125	−140
35	27	11	−4	−20	−35	−51	−67	−82	−98	−113	−129	−145
40	26	10	−6	−21	−37	−53	−69	−85	−100	−116	−132	−148
(Wind speeds greater than 40 mph have little additional effect.)	Little danger (for properly clothed person). Maximum danger of false sense of security.			Increasing danger. (Flesh may freeze within 1 minute.)			Great danger. (Flesh may freeze within 30 seconds.)					

- 215 -

Medical
Conditions

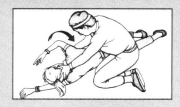

Exercise-Induced Asthma	• Also known as "exercise-induced bronchospasm."
	• Exercise-induced asthma refers to airway narrowing that occurs minutes after starting a vigorous activity. It generally peaks about 5–10 minutes after stopping the vigorous activity and usually resolves in another 20–30 minutes.
	• Many athletes have asthma.
	• Asthma episodes can be frightening, and most people are rarely well prepared to cope with them.

Exercise-Induced Asthma Care

If, during exercise, an athlete has . . .	THEN . . .
• coughing • chest tightness • wheezing when exhaling • shortness of breath • limited endurance	proceed as follows: 1. Ask if athlete has medication prescribed by a physician (usually a nebulizer). 2. Assist the athlete in taking his/her medication. 3. Some athletes may have a peak flow meter with them and know what readings indicate worsening asthma. Higher readings mean the airway is opening and asthma is getting better. Lower readings mean the airway is tightening and asthma is getting worse.

M
E
D
I
C
A
L

Exercise-Induced Asthma Care (continued)

If, during exercise, an athlete has . . .	THEN . . .
	4. If signs and symptoms get worse or don't improve within 15–30 minutes after taking the medication, then seek medical attention.

Remember: In the future, an asthmatic athlete can pretreat himself or herself by inhaling medication just before exercising and doing a gradual warm-up and cool-down.

M
E
D
I
C
A
L

Exercise-Induced Asthma Care (continued)

If the following signs appear . . .	THEN . . .
• gray or blue fingernails or lips (called cyanosis) • difficulty breathing, walking, or talking • retractions of the neck, chest, or ribs; nostrils flare • medication fails to control worsening signs and symptoms	• seek immediate medical attention by calling the EMS system • monitor the ABCs (airway, breathing, and circulation) and be prepared to give rescue breathing or CPR • pursed (narrowed) lip breathing may help reduce airway obstruction.

M
E
D
I
C
A
L

Seizures

Seizures refer to any one of several disorders caused by an abnormal electrical stimulation in the brain. Seizures may be *convulsive* or *nonconvulsive*.

Convulsive seizures involve convulsions that usually last 2–5 minutes, with complete loss of consciousness and muscle spasm.

Nonconvulsive seizures may be indicated by a blank stare lasting only a few seconds; an involuntary movement of an arm or leg; or a period of automatic movement in which awareness of one's surroundings is blurred or completely absent.

Epilepsy does not cause all seizures; they may be caused by a recent or old brain injury, a brain tumor, a stroke, high body temperature (fever), or diabetes.

Seizure Care

IF . . .	THEN . . .
• athlete has medical alert jewelry or is a known epileptic **AND** • seizures end in less than 10 minutes **AND** • consciousness returns without further incident **AND** • there are no signs of injury or physical distress	do *not* call an ambulance • place athlete on ground or floor • protect athlete's head, arms, and legs by moving objects out of the way or padding nearby objects. Do *not* rigidly restrain the athlete. • Loosen tight clothing • do *not* force anything into athlete's mouth (do *not* use a "bite stick") • do *not* put your fingers into athlete's mouth • turn athlete on side to keep airway clear after convulsions have stopped • monitor pulse and breathing

M
E
D
I
C
A
L

Seizure Care (continued)

IF . . .	THEN . . .
	• reduce athlete's embarrassment by providing privacy and having onlookers leave
	• allow the athlete to rest
	• seek medical evaluation before athlete returns to participation

Seizure Care (continued)

IF . . .	THEN . . .
• seizure happened in water • no medical alert jewelry is found, and there is no way of knowing whether the seizure is caused by epilepsy **AND** • seizure continues for more than 5 minutes • one seizure follows another with no return to full consciousness between them	• these represent medical emergencies! Call the emergency medical services (EMS) system. • place athlete on ground or floor • protect athlete's head, arms, and legs by moving objects out of the way or padding nearby objects. Do *not* rigidly restrain the athlete. • loosen tight clothing • do *not* force anything into athlete's mouth (do *not* use a "bite stick") • do *not* put your fingers into athlete's mouth • monitor pulse and breathing • turn athlete on side to keep airway clear after convulsions have stopped

M
E
D
I
C
A
L

Seizure Care (continued)

Some authorities believe that those who are seizure-prone should not participate in sports because stress or exhaustion may increase the risk of seizures. This belief is not commonly held.

Some experts believe that seizure-prone athletes should not participate in sports in which a high risk of injury is possible if a seizure were to occur (e.g., swimming, mountain climbing, hang gliding, biking, diving, and gymnastics).

When seizure-prone athletes do participate in sports, proper seizure control is mandatory.

Diabetic Emergencies	Diabetes is the inability of the body to appropriately utilize carbohydrates. The pancreas fails to produce enough of a hormone called insulin. The function of insulin is to take sugar from the blood and carry it into the body cells to be used. When excess sugar remains in the blood, the body cells must rely on fat as fuel. Since blood sugar is a major body fuel, when it cannot be used, diabetes develops.

When the blood sugar level becomes too high because of too little insulin in the blood, *diabetic coma*, or ketoacidosis, may occur. The opposite condition, *insulin shock*, can result when a person with diabetes has taken too much insulin or has not eaten. The blood sugar level drops dangerously low, and the athlete becomes weak and disoriented, or unconscious.

Both of these conditions can be fatal unless something is done to reverse them.

You may know that the athlete is diabetic; if not, look for a medical alert bracelet or necklace.

Diabetic Emergency Care

If athlete has . . .	THEN . . .
a sudden or rapid change in condition **AND** • complains of sudden hunger • displays anger or bad temper • has pale and clammy skin • staggers and displays poor coordination • appears confused or disoriented • possibly faints or becomes unconscious	suspect *insulin shock:* 1. If athlete is conscious, give sugar immediately (e.g., soft drinks, candy, or fruit juice)! Do not use diet drinks. 2. If unconscious, lay athlete on his or her side. Sprinkle some loose sugar under the tongue, because some sugar is absorbed through the mouth's lining. 3. Call the EMS system.

M
E
D
I
C
A
L

Diabetic Emergency Care (continued)

If athlete has . . .	THEN . . .
• extreme dry mouth and thirst • drowsiness • flushed, dry, and warm skin • vomiting • breath which smells fruity or like acetone (the odor of nail polish remover)	Suspect *diabetic coma* 1. Take athlete to the hospital or call the EMS system. 2. If uncertain whether the athlete is suffering from insulin shock (high blood sugar) or diabetic coma (low blood sugar), give some food or drink containing sugar.

MEDICAL

Telling the difference between the two conditions, diabetic coma and insulin shock, can be difficult. If the athlete is awake, he or she can often direct you as to what to do. If the athlete has eaten but has not taken insulin, the condition is most probably diabetic coma. If the athlete has not eaten but has taken insulin, the condition is most probably insulin shock.

If you cannot distinguish between the two conditions and sugar is available, have the athlete take it. If the condition is insulin shock, there will be a noticeable improvement. If it is diabetic coma, there is little danger that a small amount of sugar will worsen the condition. Do not give liquids to an unconscious athlete. These procedures may save the life of an athlete or avoid brain damage.

APPENDIX

A

RICE*
Procedures

Using the acronym **RICE*** helps in recalling how to properly give immediate care of musculoskeletal injuries.

For many sports injuries, **RICE** is the first aid procedure to use. It can be used for contusions (bruises), strains, sprains, dislocations, and fractures.

R = *Rest.* The first initial in the acronym **RICE** stands for rest. This means having the athlete stop moving the injured part. An injury heals faster if rested.

I = *Ice.* The second initial stands for ice or cold. An ice pack should be applied to the injured area for 20 to 30 minutes every 2 to 3 hours during the first 24 to 48 hours. The skin which is being treated with cold passes through four stages—cold, burning, aching, and numbness. When it becomes numb, remove the ice pack. This usually takes 20 to 30 minutes. After removing an ice pack, keep the part compressed with an elastic bandage and elevated (these are covered later).

Cold constricts the blood vessels to and in the injured area, which helps reduce the swelling and at the same time dulls the pain and relieves muscle spasms.

Cold should be applied as soon as possible after the injury because healing time is often directly related to the amount of swelling that occurs.

*RICE is an acronym (a word formed from the first letter or letters of each of several successive parts) for—rest, ice, compression, and elevation.

Suggested ways of applying cold to an injury:

1. *Ice bags.* Put crushed ice (or cubes) into a double plastic bag, hot water bottle, or wet towel. Apply one layer of a wet elastic bandage over the injury; place the ice pack over the injury; and then use the remaining length of elastic bandage to hold the ice pack in place. Ice bags can conform to the body's contours.

2. *Chemical "snap packs."* These sealed pouches contain two chemical envelopes that, when squeezed, mix the chemicals. A chemical reaction produces a cooling effect. Though they do not cool as well as other methods, they are convenient to use when ice is not easily available. They quickly lose their cooling power and can be used only once. They may be impractical because of expense and the danger of breakage.

Precautions when using an ice pack:

1. Do *not* apply an ice pack for more than 20 to 30 minutes at a time. Frostbite and/or nerve damage can result.

2. Do *not* place an ice pack directly on the skin. Protect the skin with a wet elastic bandage or wet towel.

3. Do *not* apply cold if the athlete has a history of circulatory disease, Raynaud's Syndrome (spasms in the arteries of the extremities that reduce circulation), abnormal sensitivity to cold, or if the injured part has been previously frostbitten.

4. Do *not* stop using an ice pack too soon. A common mistake is the early use of heat. Heat will result in swelling and pain if applied too early. Continue using an ice pack 3 to 4 times daily for the first 24 hours, and preferably up to 48 hours, before applying any heat. For severe injuries 72 hours is recommended.

5. Do *not* use a wet elastic bandage or wet towel if the athlete remains in an extremely cold environment.

C = *Compression*. The third initial, C, stands for compression. Compression of the injured area may squeeze some fluid and debris out of the injury site. In an attempt to limit internal bleeding, an elastic bandage is applied to the injured area, especially the foot, ankle, knee, thigh, hand, or elbow. An ice pack is placed over one layer of a wet elastic bandage wrap, followed by more elastic bandage applied over the ice pack to hold it in place. The ice pack, together with the elastic bandage applying compression, helps limit internal bleeding.

Use a wet elastic bandage since it will quickly transmit the cold from an ice pack to the injured area. A dry elastic bandage insulates and will not allow as much cold penetration.

Elastic bandages come in various widths—including 2- 4-, and 6-inch widths—and various lengths. Start the elastic bandage several inches below the injury and wrap in an upward, overlapping (about one-half the width of the bandage) spiral; start with an even and somewhat tight pressure, then gradually wrap more loosely above the injury.

Elastic bandages, if applied too tightly, will inhibit circulation. Therefore, stretch the elastic bandage to about 70% of its maximum length for adequate compression. Leave fingers and toes exposed to allow observation of possible change in color. Pain, pale skin, numbness, and tingling are all signs of an elastic bandage that is too tight. If any of these symptoms appear, immediately remove the elastic bandage. Leave the elastic bandage off until all the symptoms disappear; then rewrap the area, but less tightly.

Applying compression may be the most important step in preventing swelling. The athlete should wear the elastic bandage continuously for 18 to 24 hours. Although cold is applied intermittently, compression should be maintained throughout the day. At night, have the athlete loosen, but do not remove the elastic bandage.

For an ankle injury, a pad cut in the form of a "horseshoe" should be placed around the ankle knob next to the skin and under the elastic bandage in order to compress the soft tissues rather than just the bones.

E = *Elevation.* The E stands for elevation. Elevating the injured area in combination with ice packs and compression limits circulation to that area and, therefore, helps limit internal bleeding and minimize swelling.

It is simple to prop up an injured leg or arm to limit bleeding. The aim is to get the injured part above the level of the heart, whenever possible, for the first 24 hours after an injury. If a fracture is suspected, do *not* elevate an extremity until it has been stabilized with a splint. Even then, some fractures should not be elevated.

B

The Sam® Splint

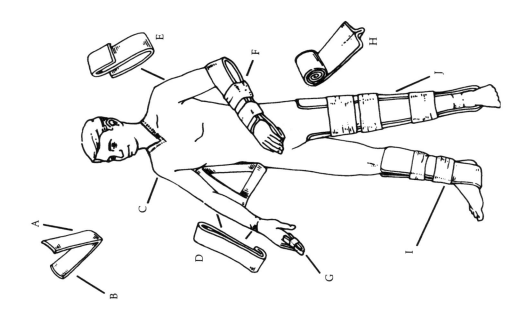

A. Fold the splint in half to create two sides. To give the splint strength, gently curve each side down the center with your thumbs.

B. This splint can be applied around the arm, forearm, or ankle and secured with kling, wrap, or roller gauze.

C. For dislocated shoulders, fold to form a triangular "Airplane" splint.

D. The splint can be doubled for increased strength.

E. The splint can be folded as above and applied to support the upper arm.

F. To splint the wrist or forearm, the splint should be applied around the elbow.

G. Sam® Finger Splints are available.

H. A T-Bend dramatically increases the strength of the splint.

I. The ankle is splinted with a single splint—folded under the foot and applied to each side.

J. Two splints can be used, one on each side of the limb, for knee or leg injuries.

Suggested First Aid Kit
Supply List

adhesive bandages (i.e., Band-Aids®, 1-inch)
adhesive tape (1- to 1-½ inch rolls)
alcohol, isopropyl (70%)
alcohol wipes
antibiotic ointment (i.e., Polysporin™, Neosporin™)
antifungal cream (i.e., Tinactin™, Micatin™)
chemical cold "snap packs"
coin money for pay telephone
cotton tip applicators (i.e., Q–tips®)
disinfectant, skin (Betadine®)
disinfecting soap (i.e., pHisoHex)
disposable gloves (latex)
elastic bandages/wraps (i.e., Ace® bandage, both
    3- and 4-inch widths)
emergency information cards completed for all athletes
emergency telephone numbers
face mask, one-way valve
felt (both ½-inch and ¼-inch thick, 6- by 6-inch square)
flashlight or penlight

gauze pads, sterile (both 2- and 4-inch sizes)
gauze roller bandages, self-adhering, sterile (2-, 3-,
    and 4-inch sizes) (i.e., Kerlix, Kling®)
moleskin (6- by 10-inch size)
non-stick gauze pads (i.e., Telfa® pads, 3- by 4-inch size)
paper drinking cups
pencil and paper
petroleum jelly (i.e., Vaseline®)
plastic bags for ice
powder, talcum and/or foot powder
scissors—bandage and biological
Spenco Second Skin™
splints (i.e., Sam® Splint)
sunscreen (15 + SPF)
thermometers (rectal and oral)
tongue depressors
triangular bandages
tweezers

Place items in a brightly colored fishing tackle box or tool box marked as a first aid kit for storage and transporting.

This first aid kit is for sports and athletic situations. Other situations—such as backpacking, home, motor vehicle, and work—dictate other items for a first aid kit.

Bones of the Body

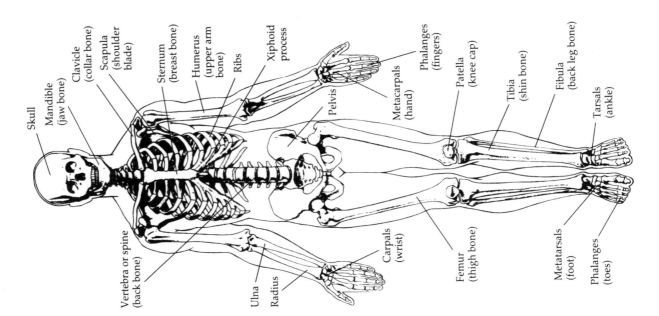

Skull

Mandible (jaw bone)

Clavicle (collar bone)

Scapula (shoulder blade)

Sternum (breast bone)

Humerus (upper arm bone)

Ribs

Xiphoid process

Pelvis

Metacarpals (hand)

Phalanges (fingers)

Patella (knee cap)

Tibia (shin bone)

Fibula (back leg bone)

Tarsals (ankle)

Vertebra or spine (back bone)

Ulna

Radius

Carpals (wrist)

Femur (thigh bone)

Metatarsals (foot)

Phalanges (toes)

E

Major Muscle Groups
of the Body

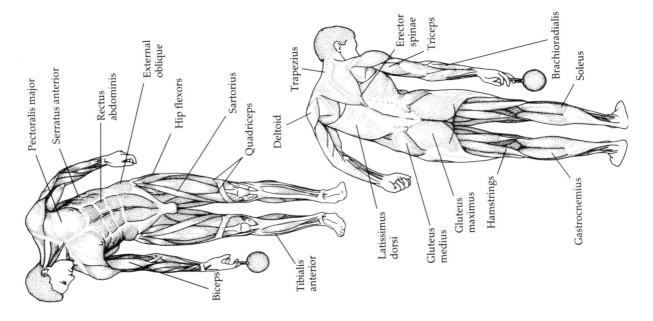

Pectoralis major
Serratus anterior
Rectus abdominis
External oblique
Hip flexors
Sartorius
Quadriceps
Biceps
Tibialis anterior

Trapezius
Deltoid
Erector spinae
Triceps
Brachioradialis
Soleus
Latissimus dorsi
Gluteus medius
Gluteus maximus
Hamstrings
Gastrocnemius